D0690288

Advanced Concepts of

Personal
Training
Lab Manual
SECOND EDITION

Brian Biagioli, Ed.D

University of Miami

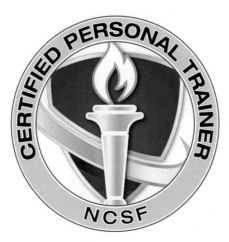

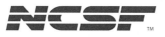

NATIONAL COUNCIL ON
STRENGTH & FITNESS

Contributing Authors

Arturo Leyva, PhD

Davy Levy, MS

Jennifer Maher, PhD

Lafayette Watson, PhD

Robert Silver, MS

Craig Flanagan, PhD

Steven Hicks, MS

Sean Grieve, MS

Steven Wermus, MS

Ozgur Alan, PhD

Taylor Snook, MS

ISBN: 978-0-9791696-9-4

Copyright © 2019 National Council on Strength & Fitness (NCSF)

All rights reserved. Except for use in a review, the reproduction or utilization of this work in any form or by any electronic, mechanical, or other means, now known or hereafter invented, including xerography, photocopying, and recording, and in any information retrieval system, is forbidden without the written permission of the National Council on Strength & Fitness.

Printed in the United States of America

Our printing requirements use a mix of recycled and environmentally sustainable (FSC and COC) papers.

Distributed by:

National Council on Strength & Fitness

5915 Ponce de Leon Blvd., Suite 60

Coral Gables, FL 33146

800-772-NCSF(6273)

www.NCSF.org

Table of Contents

◆ Movement Application

This lab corresponds to Chapter 2: pages 26-29 and 48-65

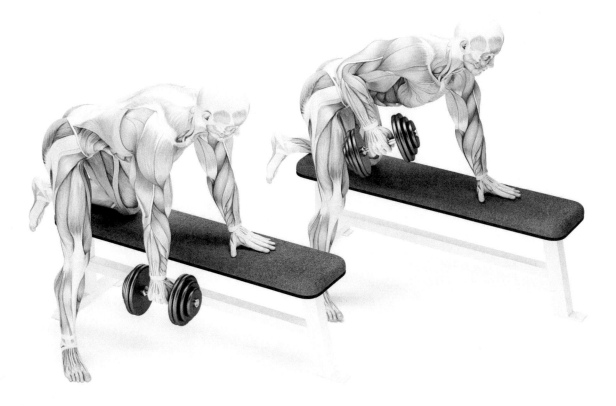

Activity 1   Skeletal and Muscular Structure Identification

Activity Description

A step in understanding human movement and how it relates to exercise is being able to properly identify specific anatomical structures of the body. The following section contains illustrations of the human axial and appendicular skeletal systems and associated muscular anatomy. As a personal trainer, you will be expected to recognize anatomical terms and apply these terms to describe specific bodily movements.

Procedures

Using the terms provided, correctly label the following anatomical structures. You may refer to Chapter 2 of your course textbook to assist you.

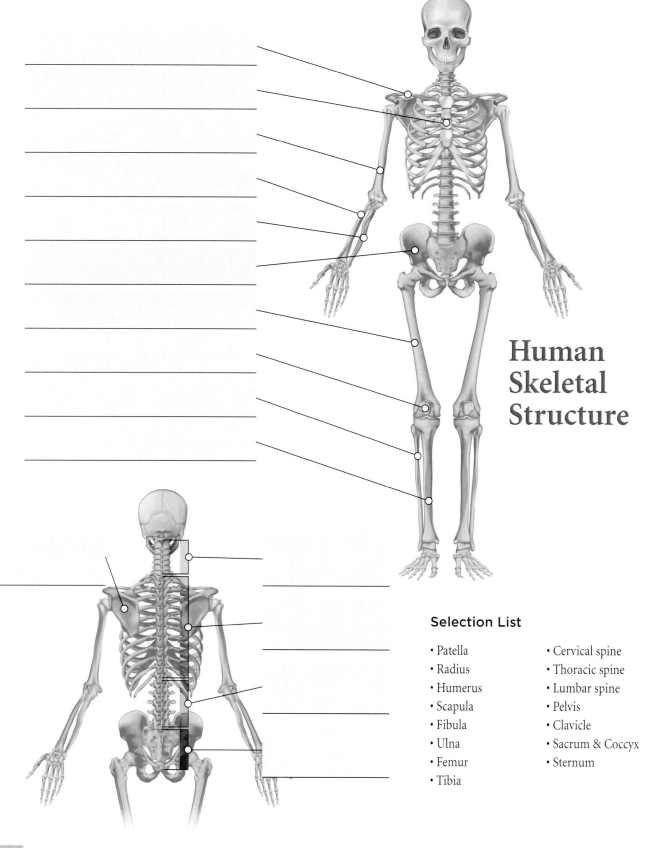

Human Skeletal Structure

Selection List

- Patella
- Radius
- Humerus
- Scapula
- Fibula
- Ulna
- Femur
- Tibia
- Cervical spine
- Thoracic spine
- Lumbar spine
- Pelvis
- Clavicle
- Sacrum & Coccyx
- Sternum

Upper Body Anterior View

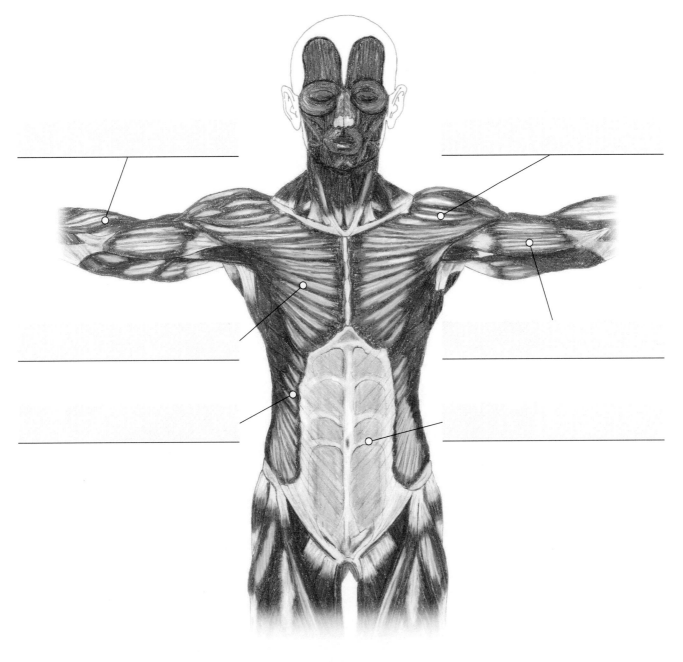

Selection List
- Rectus Abdominis
- Pectoralis Major
- Deltoid
- Biceps Brachii
- Brachioradialis
- External Oblique

Upper Body Posterior View

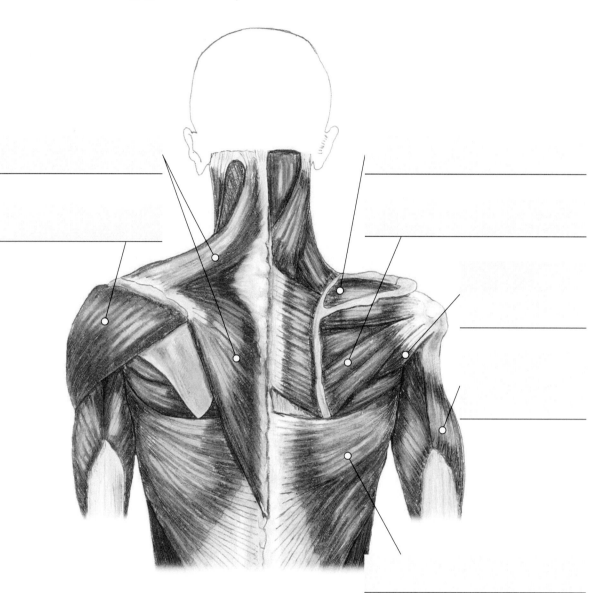

Selection List
- Teres Minor
- Infraspinatus
- Supraspinatus
- Deltoid
- Trapezius
- Latissimus Dorsi
- Triceps Brachii

Lower Body Anterior View

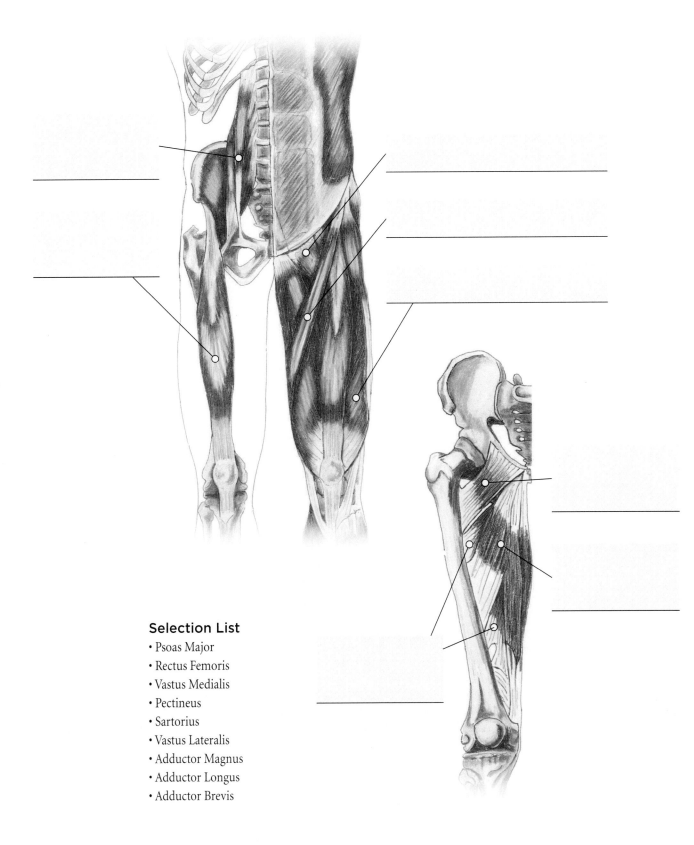

Selection List
- Psoas Major
- Rectus Femoris
- Vastus Medialis
- Pectineus
- Sartorius
- Vastus Lateralis
- Adductor Magnus
- Adductor Longus
- Adductor Brevis

Lower Body Posterior View

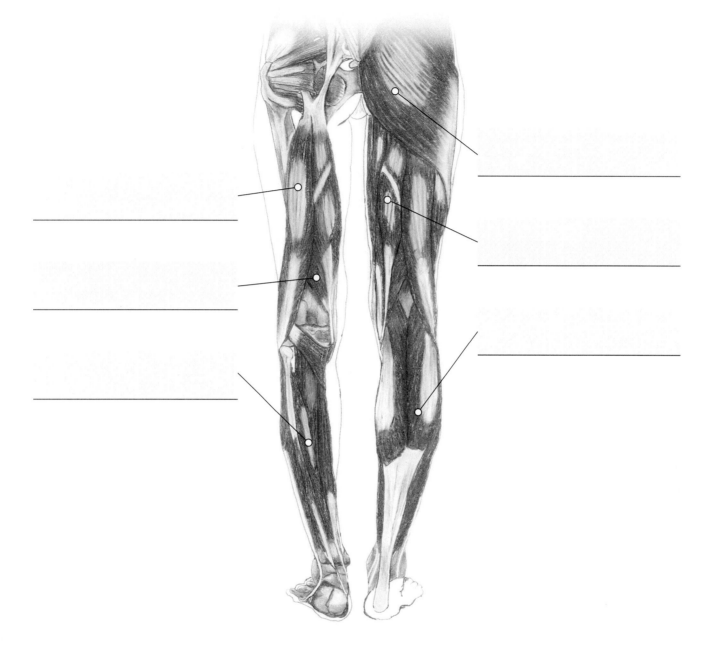

Selection List
- Gluteus Maximus
- Semitendinosus
- Biceps Femoris
- Semimembranosus
- Soleus
- Gastrocnemius

Activity 2 Movement Descriptions

Activity Description

Anatomists have developed a specific vocabulary to describe anatomical movements, identify the position of anatomical structures and describe muscle function as it relates to movement. Some of these terms are widely employed in exercise science and fitness training environments. It is important that you become familiar with the working definitions of these terms, particularly as they relate to human movement and exercise.

Procedures

In the spaces provided identify and label the pelvic position demonstrated in the illustrations.

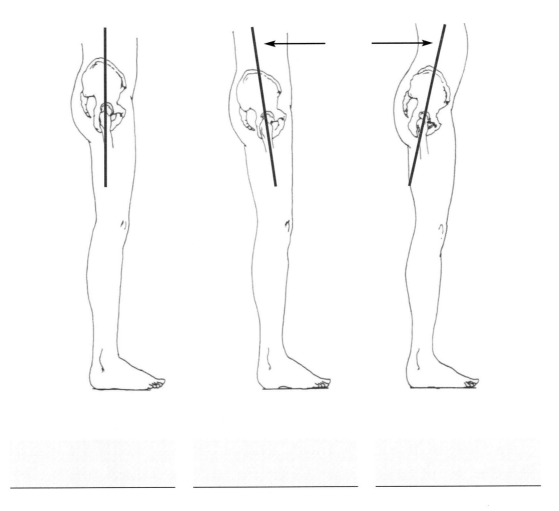

_____   _____   _____

Procedures

Identify the joint action, prime mover(s) and assistive mover(s) for each of the following illustrated movements. Then provide a common exercise used in resistance training associated with the movement.

Glenohumeral (Shoulder) Joint

Flexion

Muscles Involved: _____

Common Exercise: _____

Extension

Muscles Involved: _____

Common Exercise: _____

Adduction

Muscles Involved: _____

Common Exercise: _____

Abduction

Muscles Involved: _____

Common Exercise: _____

Horizontal Adduction

Muscles Involved: _____

Common Exercise: _____

Horizontal Abduction

Muscles Involved: _____

Common Exercise: _____

Internal Rotation

Muscles Involved: _____

Common Exercise: _____

External Rotation

Muscles Involved: _____

Common Exercise: _____

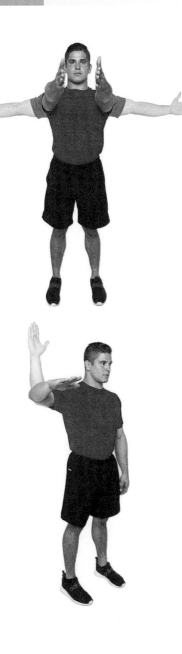

Elbows

Flexion

Muscles Involved: _____

Common Exercise: _____

Extension

Muscles Involved: _____

Common Exercise: _____

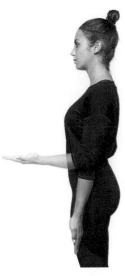

Trunk and Spine

Flexion

Muscles Involved: _____

Common Exercise: _____

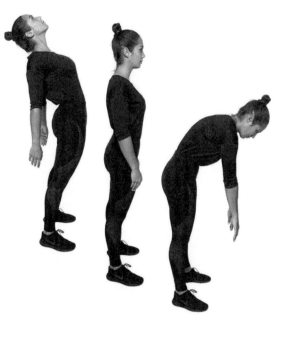

Extension

Muscles Involved: _____

Common Exercise: _____

Lateral Flexion / Abduction

Muscles Involved: _____

Common Exercise: _____

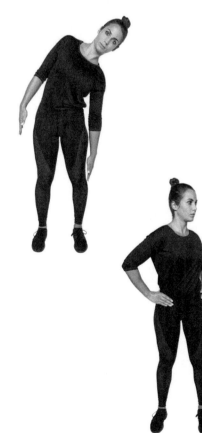

Rotation

Muscles Involved: _____

Common Exercise: _____

Movement Application

Hips

Flexion

Muscles Involved: _____

Common Exercise: _____

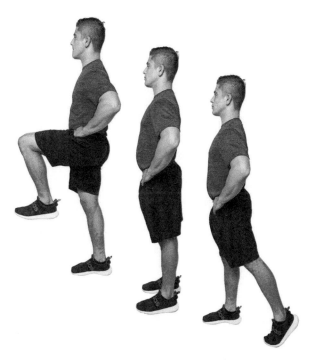

Extension

Muscles Involved: _____

Common Exercise: _____

Adduction

Muscles Involved: _____

Common Exercise: _____

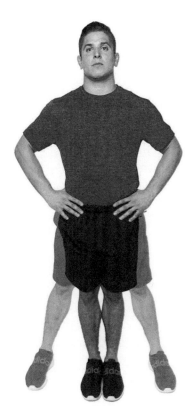

Abduction

Muscles Involved: _____

Common Exercise: _____

Knees

Flexion

Muscles Involved: _____

Common Exercise: _____

Extension

Muscles Involved: _____

Common Exercise: _____

Ankles

Plantarflexion

Muscles Involved: _____

Common Exercise: _____

Dorsiflexion

Muscles Involved: _____

Common Exercise: _____

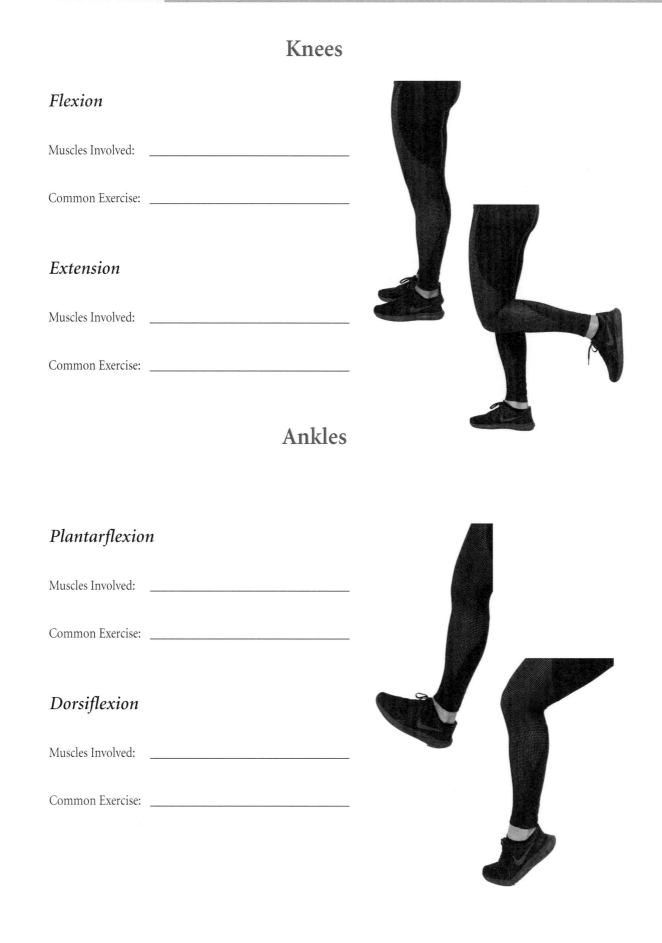

Activity 3 **Anatomical Planes**

Activity Description

Once the structures of the body can be identified and a working knowledge of the previous anatomical terms has been established, these terms can be applied to planes of movement. This will allow for a complete description of any number of actions. An anatomical plane is an imaginary, flat, two-dimensional surface that divides the body into various segments. Anatomical planes help describe positions, relationships, and directions of movement by the human body. When more than one plane is used, as is common in multi-joint exercises, the direction of the center of mass is commonly used to identify the primary plane.

Procedures

Fill in the appropriate plane in the spaces provided. Refer to Chapter 2 of your textbook as needed.

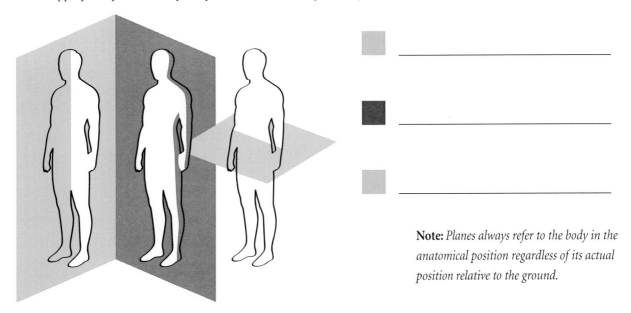

Note: *Planes always refer to the body in the anatomical position regardless of its actual position relative to the ground.*

Identify the movement plane(s) by which each of the following exercises occur.

Bicep curl: _____

Box step-up: _____

DB shoulder press: _____

Barbell back squat: _____

Lat pull-down: _____

Romanian deadlift: _____

Lunge with rotation: _____

Movement Application Lab Quiz

1. What group of muscles does the pectineus participate with for movement and stability?

    _____ a. Hip adductors
    _____ b. Hip abductors
    _____ c. Ankle flexors
    _____ d. Spinal flexors

2. What portion of the spine is most functionally affected by tilts of the pelvis?

    _____ a. Thoracic
    _____ b. Cervical
    _____ c. Lumbar
    _____ d. Sacrum

3. Which of the following arm bones would not move during proper performance of a biceps curl?

    _____ a. Radius
    _____ b. Ulna
    _____ c. Humerus
    _____ d. Tibia

4. Which of the following muscles internally rotates shoulder joints?

    _____ a. Supraspinatus
    _____ b. Subscapularis
    _____ c. Infraspinatus
    _____ d. Teres minor

5. Which of the following is the prime mover during shoulder flexion?

    _____ a. Latissimus dorsi
    _____ b. Trapezius
    _____ c. Deltoid
    _____ d. Rhomboids

6. Which body segment can laterally flex?

___ a. Ankle
___ b. Shoulder
___ c. Pelvis
___ d. Spine

7. Which of the following would be activated to extend the spine during a good morning exercise?

___ a. Rectus abdominis
___ b. Quadratus lumborum
___ c. Rectus femoris
___ d. Erector spinae

8. Which of the following muscles is associated with movements involving the ankle?

___ a. Gastrocnemius
___ b. Semitendinosus
___ c. Multifidus
___ d. Biceps femoris

9. Which of the following exercises is performed in the frontal plane?

___ a. Modified deadlift
___ b. Triceps extension
___ c. Cable trunk rotation
___ d. Lateral lunge

10. Which of the following combination exercises involves a single primary movement plane?

___ a. Lunge with MB rotation
___ b. Step-up with DB lateral raise
___ c. Reverse lunge with cable row
___ d. All of the above are multi-planar

Movement Application

◆ Resistance Training Techniques

This lab corresponds to the following text/content – Chapter 2: Pages 66-109
(Please also review E-learning videos prior to participation in this lab)

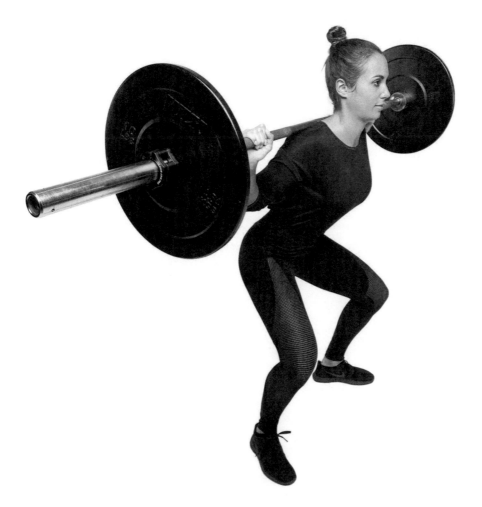

Lab Description

Resistance training is a vital component in the development of total fitness and function. The effects of participating in a regular resistance training program are far-reaching, aiding in proper posture, enhancement of joint/bone health, improved movement economy, improved body composition, maintenance of proper function and independence, and decreasing the rate of muscle loss associated with aging (sarcopenia). As a competent exercise professional, you must be able to understand the physiological effects of resistance training to the degree that you can explain the important benefits of this mode of exercise to clients. Additionally, key job tasks include: 1) competently designing and implementing a resistance training program based on client-specific goals, capabilities, and needs, 2) identifying, explaining, and demonstrating the correct biomechanical execution of resistance training exercises, 3) identifying appropriate starting points and instructing efficient skill acquisition and progressions, and 4) effectively utilizing the principles of specificity, overload, progression, and periodization.

Activity 1   **Upper Body Resistance Training**

Activity Description

The exercises presented are intended to give a foundation for upper body resistance training. Although there are numerous exercises and variations that can be utilized, the exercises performed cover primary actions of the upper body musculature. Consistent with most resistance-based activities, many of these movements can also be performed using various resistance modalities (e.g., barbells, dumbbells, machines, tubing, cables, medicine balls, etc.).

Procedures

Have a volunteer subject/partner perform the following exercises under your guidance and supervision. Read the activity description in Chapter 2 of the course textbook and have a thorough understanding of each movement prior to performance of the exercise. At the completion of this activity, participants should be able to properly describe, demonstrate, instruct, and spot each activity for all clients. Instructors should use the check-off box to indicate successful completion of the exercise.

Example

Barbell Bench Press

Primary Joint Action:	Humeral horizontal adduction, elbow extension
Primary Muscles Involved:	Pectoralis major, anterior deltoid, triceps brachii
Common Errors:	Improper deceleration to chest, hip extension
Spotting Technique:	Assisted lift-off, spot the bar, re-rack with alternate grip

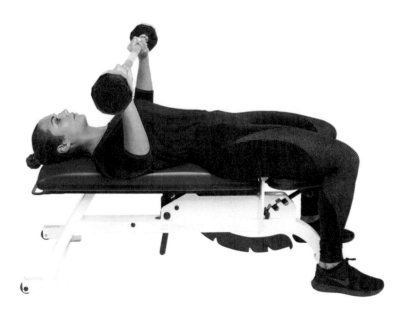

DB Chest Press *(page 68)*

Primary Joint Action: _____

_____

Primary Muscles Involved: _____

_____

Common Errors: _____

_____

Spotting Technique: _____

_____

☐ Activity Performed

Incline Bench Press *(page 69)*

Primary Joint Action: _____

_____

Primary Muscles Involved: _____

_____

Common Errors: _____

_____

Spotting Technique: _____

_____

☐ Activity Performed

Chest Fly *(page 70)*

Primary Joint Action: _____

_____

Primary Muscles Involved: _____

_____

Common Errors: _____

_____

Spotting Technique: _____

_____

☐ Activity Performed

Bench Push-up *(page 71)*

Primary Joint Action: _____

_____

Primary Muscles Involved: _____

_____

Common Errors: _____

_____

☐ Activity Performed

Military Press *(page 72)*

Primary Joint Action: _____

_____

Primary Muscles Involved: _____

_____

Common Errors: _____

_____

Spotting Technique: _____

_____

☐ Activity Performed

Dumbbell Shoulder Press *(page 73)*

Primary Joint Action: _____

_____

Primary Muscles Involved: _____

_____

Common Errors: _____

_____

Spotting Technique: _____

_____

☐ Activity Performed

DB Upright Row *(page 74)*

Primary Joint Action: _____

_____

Primary Muscles Involved: _____

_____

Common Errors: _____

_____

☐ Activity Performed

Lateral Deltoid Raise *(page 75)*

Primary Joint Action: _____

_____

Primary Muscles Involved: _____

_____

Common Errors: _____

_____

Spotting Technique: _____

_____

☐ Activity Performed

Rear Deltoid Raise *(page 76)*

Primary Joint Action: _____

_____

Primary Muscles Involved: _____

_____

Common Errors: _____

_____

Spotting Technique: _____

_____

☐ Activity Performed

Front Raise *(page 77)*

Primary Joint Action: _____

_____

Primary Muscles Involved: _____

_____

Common Errors: _____

_____

☐ Activity Performed

Bent-Over Row *(page 78)*

Primary Joint Action: _____

_____

Primary Muscles Involved: _____

_____

Common Errors: _____

_____

☐ Activity Performed

Single-Arm Row *(page 79)*

Primary Joint Action: _____

_____

Primary Muscles Involved: _____

_____

Common Errors: _____

_____

☐ Activity Performed

Seated Row *(page 80)*

Primary Joint Action: _____

_____

Primary Muscles Involved: _____

_____

Common Errors: _____

_____

☐ Activity Performed

Lat Pull-down *(page 81)*

Primary Joint Action: _____

_____

Primary Muscles Involved: _____

_____

Common Errors: _____

_____

Spotting Technique: _____

_____

☐ Activity Performed

Triceps Extension *(page 82)*

Primary Joint Action: _____

_____

Primary Muscles Involved: _____

_____

Common Errors: _____

_____

Spotting Technique: _____

_____

☐ Activity Performed

Triceps Kickback *(page 83)*

Primary Joint Action: _____

_____

Primary Muscles Involved: _____

_____

Common Errors: _____

_____

Spotting Technique: _____

_____

☐ Activity Performed

Triceps Push-down *(page 84)*

Primary Joint Action: _____

_____

Primary Muscles Involved: _____

_____

Common Errors: _____

_____

☐ Activity Performed

Bicep Curl *(page 85)*

Primary Joint Action: _____

_____

Primary Muscles Involved: _____

_____

Common Errors: _____

_____

Spotting Technique: _____

_____

☐ Activity Performed

Hammer Curls *(page 86)*

Primary Joint Action: _____

_____

Primary Muscles Involved: _____

_____

Common Errors: _____

_____

Spotting Technique: _____

_____

☐ Activity Performed

Upper Body Resistance Training Quiz

1. Which of the following is the primary muscle involved during the incline barbell press?

    _____ a. Biceps
    _____ b. Pectoralis major
    _____ c. Rhomboids
    _____ d. Posterior deltoids

2. Where should the trainer spot the dumbbell chest press exercise?

    _____ a. At the dumbbells
    _____ b. At the elbows
    _____ c. At the wrists
    _____ d. At the shoulders

3. Which of the following exercises involve shoulder horizontal abduction?

    _____ a. Bicep curls
    _____ b. Dumbbell shoulder press
    _____ c. Lat pull-down
    _____ d. Bent-over row

4. Which of the following concerning the military press is correct?

    _____ a. The lift can be performed behind the head for greater deltoid activation
    _____ b. Flexing the hips during the eccentric phase helps maintain proper form
    _____ c. Spotting should occur at the distal end of each humerus when standing
    _____ d. Engaging a slight backward lean will help properly activate the latissimus dorsi

5. A _____ grip is favorable during frontal raises as this lowers the risk for injury and potentially increases the range of motion.

    _____ a. Neutral
    _____ b. Pronated
    _____ c. Supinated
    _____ d. Alternating

6. All of the following are primary muscles involved during the single-arm row, except:

_____ a. Rhomboids
_____ b. Brachioradialis
_____ c. Latissimus dorsi
_____ d. Anterior deltoid

7. Which of the following statements concerning the seated cable row is correct?

_____ a. A common error is to perform arm flexion at the expense of scapular retraction
_____ b. The client should lean forward in between repetitions to generate momentum
_____ c. The exercise is spotted at the trunk, just above the hips
_____ d. An anterior pelvic tilt is performed during the entire movement to maintain spinal stability

8. Which of the following exercises loses activation effectiveness when performed using dumbbells versus cable or band resistance?

_____ a. Overhead presses
_____ b. Triceps kickbacks
_____ c. Hammer curls
_____ d. Rows

9. What is the correct movement of the shoulder during the standing tricep cable push-down?

_____ a. Extension
_____ b. Flexion
_____ c. Internal rotation
_____ d. No movement

10. Which of the following exercises can be spotted at the wrist or forearm?

_____ a. Dumbbell upright row
_____ b. Dumbbell chest fly
_____ c. Military press
_____ d. Lat pull-down

Activity 2 **Lower Body Resistance Training**

Activity Description

This activity presents traditional lower body resistance training exercise techniques. A progressive continuum exists for each exercise, which enables the exercise professional to manipulate movements to fit the individual abilities of different clients. The goal of this lab is to focus on the proper instruction of exercise form and technique. If an individual cannot perform an exercise correctly, a modification can be made, or a different exercise can be substituted in its place. Body alignment and mechanics are vital to safe and effective execution of movements under resistance. This makes recognizing and controlling proper body movements a pivotal skill for the exercise professional and should be a primary consideration in this lab experience. Practicing the activities without weight or with very little resistance at the onset of the instruction will enable the subject to develop correct motor patterning and enhanced kinesthetic awareness. Skill acquisition and progressions should follow a building-block approach to best acclimate the body for the next task. Using appropriate teaching cues and hands-on instruction will aid in the learning process. Joint alignment is particularly important with resistance training and should be closely monitored during each exercise.

Procedures

Have a volunteer subject/partner perform the following exercises under your guidance and supervision. Be sure to read the activity description in Chapter 2 of the course textbook and have a thorough understanding of each movement prior to the performance of the exercise. ***Remember, viewing the E-learning videos for these exercises before execution is preferred.*** This is of extreme importance as exercise professionals must have a comprehensive working knowledge of a multitude of training techniques and be able to properly describe, demonstrate, instruct, and spot each activity for new and veteran clients. Upon completion of this activity, participants should be able to properly describe, demonstrate, instruct, and spot each exercise. Instructors should use the check-off box to indicate successful completion of the exercise.

Example

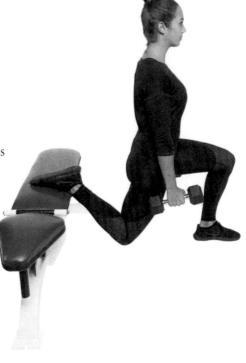

Single-leg 'Bulgarian' Squat

Primary Joint Action:
Hip extension, knee extension

Primary Muscles Involved:
Gluteus maximus, rectus femoris, bicep femoris, vastus intermedius

Common Errors:
Knee crosses plane of toe, incomplete back leg flexion

Back Squat *(page 87-88)*

Primary Joint Action: _____

_____

Primary Muscles Involved: _____

_____

Common Errors: _____

_____

Spotting Technique: _____

_____

☐ Activity Performed

Front Squat *(page 89-90)*

Primary Joint Action: _____

_____

Primary Muscles Involved: _____

_____

Common Errors: _____

_____

Spotting Technique: _____

_____

☐ Activity Performed

Traditional Deadlift *(page 91)*

Primary Joint Action: _____

_____

Primary Muscles Involved: _____

_____

Common Errors: _____

_____

☐ Activity Performed

Modified Deadlift *(page 92)*

Primary Joint Action: _____

_____

Primary Muscles Involved: _____

_____

Common Errors: _____

_____

☐ Activity Performed

Romanian Deadlift *(page 93)*

Primary Joint Action: _____

_____

Primary Muscles Involved: _____

_____

Common Errors: _____

_____

☐ Activity Performed

Lunge *(page 94)*

Primary Joint Action: _____

_____

Primary Muscles Involved: _____

_____

Common Errors: _____

_____

☐ Activity Performed

Resistance Training Techniques

Lateral Lunge *(page 95)*

Primary Joint Action: _____

_____

Primary Muscles Involved: _____

_____

Common Errors: _____

_____

☐ Activity Performed

Step-up *(page 96)*

Primary Joint Action: _____

_____

Primary Muscles Involved: _____

_____

Common Errors: _____

_____

☐ Activity Performed

Physioball Leg Curl *(page 98)*

Primary Joint Action: _____

_____

Primary Muscles Involved: _____

_____

Common Errors: _____

_____

Spotting Technique: _____

_____

☐ Activity Performed

Heel Raise *(page 99)*

Primary Joint Action: _____

_____

Primary Muscles Involved: _____

_____

Common Errors: _____

_____

☐ Activity Performed

Lower Body Resistance Training Quiz

1. Where is the proper spotting location during a barbell back squat?

   ____ a. Just above the hips
   ____ b. On the barbell
   ____ c. On the chest
   ____ d. Outside of the ribcage

2. Which of the following is primary muscle group trained during the front squat?

   ____ a. Quadriceps
   ____ b. Hamstrings
   ____ c. Abductors
   ____ d. Calves

3. What is the correct biomechanical cue for the traditional deadlift?

   ____ a. Start with the back parallel to the ground
   ____ b. Extending the knees, hips and trunk at the same rate
   ____ c. Lean back to put the weight on the heels
   ____ d. Keep the bar against the shins during the concentric phase

4. All of the following should be verbally and physical cued rather than directly spotted, except:

   ____ a. Romanian deadlift
   ____ b. Step-up
   ____ c. Front squat
   ____ d. Lateral lunge

5. Squats and deadlifts are performed in the _____ plane?

   ____ a. Sagittal
   ____ b. Frontal
   ____ c. Transverse
   ____ d. Ipsilateral

6. Which of the following exercises is used to stretch the hip flexors?

_____ a. Back squats
_____ b. Single-leg (Bulgarian) squat
_____ c. Modified deadlift
_____ d. Physioball leg curl

7. Which of the following is correct concerning a dumbbell lunge?

_____ a. The knees can cross the toes to attain full ROM
_____ b. Small steps should be taken to keep proper hip-knee alignment
_____ c. The reverse lunge is hip muscle dominant
_____ d. The spine should migrate forward to place greater emphasis on the quadriceps

8. Which exercise emphasizes the hamstrings as the prime mover group:

_____ a. Single-leg squat
_____ b. Lateral lunge
_____ c. Forward lunge
_____ d. Romanian deadlift

9. During performance of a seated calf raise, _____ activation is emphasized.

_____ a. Gastrocnemius
_____ b. Peroneus brevis
_____ c. Soleus
_____ d. Anterior tibialis

10. All of the following are true concerning a physioball leg curl, except:

_____ a. Spotting is provided at the ball as needed
_____ b. The ankles and femurs should remain neutral
_____ c. The hips should remain flexed at all times to maximize hamstring activation
_____ d. The exercise primarily involves activation of the biceps femoris

Activity 3 **Trunk Musculature Resistance Training**

Activity Description

The exercises presented within this activity are intended to give the user a foundation for resistance training movements for the trunk musculature. Although there are numerous variations that can be utilized in a program, the exercises provided cover the primary actions of the trunk including flexion, extension, lateral flexion, and rotation. Many of the movements can be performed using various resistance modalities (e.g., barbells, dumbbells, machines, tubing, cables, medicine balls, etc.), but for all intended purposes, there is little variation in the gross mechanical execution of each exercise regardless of the resistance used.

Procedures

Have a volunteer subject/partner perform the following resistance training exercises under your guidance and supervision. Be sure to read the activity descriptions in Chapter 2 of the course textbook and have a thorough understanding of each movement prior to the performance of the exercise. *Remember, viewing the E-learning videos for these exercises before execution is preferred.* Upon completion of this activity, participants should be able to properly describe, demonstrate, instruct, and spot each activity for new and experienced clients. Instructors should use the check-off box to indicate successful completion of the exercise.

Example

Cable Rotation

Primary Joint Action:
Trunk rotation

Primary Muscles Involved:
Obliques

Common Errors:
Shoulder movement, knee/hip rotation

Abdominal Curl-up *(page 100)*

Primary Joint Action: _____

_____

Primary Muscles Involved: _____

_____

Common Errors: _____

_____

☐ Activity Performed

Reverse Abdominal Curl-up *(page 101)*

Primary Joint Action: _____

_____

Primary Muscles Involved: _____

_____

Common Errors: _____

_____

☐ Activity Performed

Alternating Ankle Touches *(page 102)*

Primary Joint Action: _____

_____

Primary Muscles Involved: _____

_____

Common Errors: _____

_____

☐ Activity Performed

Floor Bridging *(page 103)*

Primary Joint Action: _____

_____

Primary Muscles Involved: _____

_____

Common Errors: _____

_____

☐ Activity Performed

Opposite Raises *(page 104)*

Primary Joint Action: _____

_____

Primary Muscles Involved: _____

_____

Common Errors: _____

_____

☐ Activity Performed

Goodmorning *(page 105)*

Primary Joint Action: _____

_____

Primary Muscles Involved: _____

_____

Common Errors: _____

_____

☐ Activity Performed

Physioball Roll-up *(page 106)*

Primary Joint Action: _____

_____

Primary Muscles Involved: _____

_____

Common Errors: _____

_____

☐ Activity Performed

Medicine Ball Chops *(page 107)*

Primary Joint Action: _____

_____

Primary Muscles Involved: _____

_____

Common Errors: _____

_____

☐ Activity Performed

Medicine Ball Rotation Pass *(page 108)*

Primary Joint Action: _____

_____

Primary Muscles Involved: _____

_____

Common Errors: _____

_____

☐ Activity Performed

Medicine Ball Pullover *(page 109)*

Primary Joint Action: _____

_____

Primary Muscles Involved: _____

_____

Common Errors: _____

_____

☐ Activity Performed

Trunk Musculature Resistance Training Quiz

1. Trunk flexion is a primary joint action during all of the following, except:

    ____ a. Abdominal curl-up
    ____ b. Floor bridging
    ____ c. Reverse abdominal curl-up
    ____ d. Physioball roll-up

2. Which of the following will stretch the hamstrings to the greatest degree?

    ____ a. Opposite raises
    ____ b. Abdominal curl-ups
    ____ c. Goodmorning
    ____ d. Medicine ball chops

3. Which of the following does not involve the rectus abdominis as a primary mover?

    ____ a. Physioball roll-up
    ____ b. Medicine ball chops
    ____ c. Medicine ball pullover
    ____ d. Opposite raises

4. Which of the following would be the best choice for activating the internal and external obliques?

    ____ a. Medicine ball pullover
    ____ b. Medicine ball rotation pass
    ____ c. Medicine ball chops
    ____ d. Floor bridging

5. Which of the following is true concerning reverse abdominal curl-ups?

    ____ a. The hip angle should remain constant to ensure proper activation
    ____ b. The most common error is excess knee flexion
    ____ c. The pelvis should remain neutral
    ____ d. The gluteals should remain on the ground at all times

6. Shoulder stability is heavily challenged during _____ ?

        ____   a.   Medicine ball pullovers
        ____   b.   Physioball roll-ups
        ____   c.   MB rotation passes
        ____   d.   Alternating ankle touches

7. What is a common error when performing a MB rotation pass?

        ____   a.   Rotating the hip
        ____   b.   Excess shoulder action
        ____   c.   Excess foot movement
        ____   d.   All the above

8. Which exercise activates the glutes as a prime mover?

        ____   a.   Physioball roll-ups
        ____   b.   Alternating ankle touches
        ____   c.   Opposite raise
        ____   d.   Reverse curl up

9. In what exercise does the ball rebound material matter due to safety?

        ____   a.   MB pullover
        ____   b.   MB chop
        ____   c.   MB rotation pass
        ____   d.   All the above

10. What exercise requires active back extension?

        ____   a.   Physioball roll-ups
        ____   b.   Alternating ankle touches
        ____   c.   Floor bridge
        ____   d.   Reverse curl up

◆ Human Physiology Applications

This lab corresponds to the following text – Chapter 4: Pages 142-155, 167-174

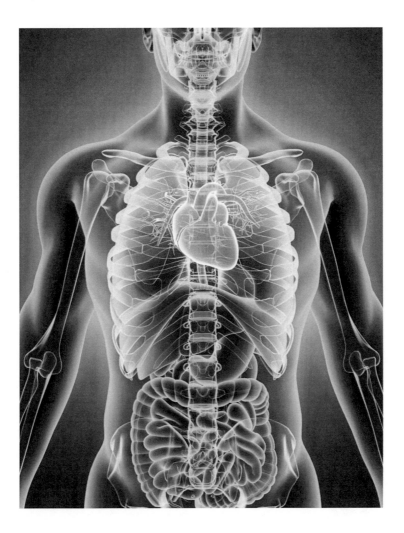

Activity 1   Anaerobic Power Step Test

Activity Description

The metabolic systems of the body are designed to meet specific demands. The duration of time and intensity by which the activity is performed ultimately determines the energy system contribution. When the intensity is elevated, and prolonged, different energy systems attempt to maximize ATP production to support force output requirements, but each system has limits to this production.

The anaerobic power step test forces the body to work within the phosphagen system and glycolytic pathways. The decline in force output can be tracked by identifying shifts in contribution from each system. The assessment lasts for 60 seconds, which enables it to measure both short- and long-term anaerobic power. Energy requirements are primarily dependent upon the glycolytic pathway of anaerobic metabolism with secondary support from the phosphagen energy system. Due to the length and intensity of the test, significant lactate production (muscle acidity) can be expected. It is somewhat isolated from general circulation because only one leg is used for the test. This test is an excellent example of the body's response to high-intensity anaerobic training reflected by a concurrent decline in movement speed with an increase in heart and respiration rates in response to changing muscle pH levels.

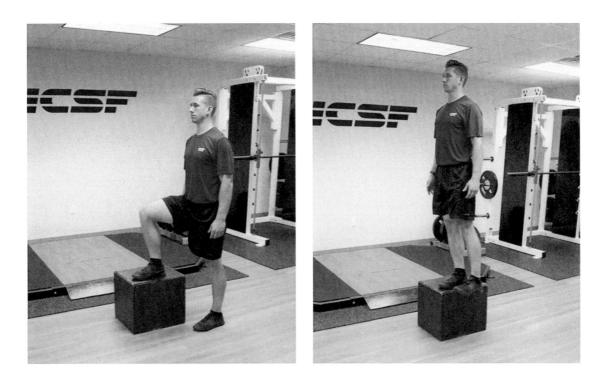

Equipment

- Step or box
- Stopwatch

Procedures

Step 1 **Start Position:** The subject should stand alongside a 16-inch box or step. Note: If a different height box or step is employed it changes the 0.4 m standard in the formula.

Step 2 The subject starts with the foot of their dominant leg (testing leg) centered on top of the step. The (step) foot will remain in the same location throughout the duration of the test.

Step 3 **Start Test:** On the "Go" command, the timer starts, and the subject begins the step-up. On each step, the subject's legs and back should be straightened with the arms remaining at the sides of the body.

Step 4 The subject should attempt to move as fast as possible through the full range of motion (ROM). Tests should not be paced but performed at an all-out exertion for the entire duration (60 seconds).

Step 5 **Scoring:** A step is counted each time the subject's step leg is straightened and then returned to the starting position. Steps are not counted if the subject does not straighten the step leg or if the subject's hip is flexed.

Step 6 The tester should call out the time remaining every 15 seconds. The total number of steps should be recorded for the 60-second trial.

Step 7 **Stop Test:** At the end of the 60-second period, the trainer should stop the test and record the total number of steps.

Number of Steps Completed _____

Step 8 Have the subject perform a cool down to prevent blood pooling in the working leg.

How to Calculate

Anaerobic Capacity (kgm · min^{-1}) = {_____ kg x [(0.4 m × _____ step score)/1]} × 1.33

= [_____ kg × (_____) m / 1] × 1.33

= _____ kg × _____ m · min^{-1} × 1.33

= _____ (kgm · min^{-1})

Watts = _____ (kgm · min^{-1}) ÷ 6.12 W/ kgm · m^{-1}

Example

An 80 kg (176 lbs.) male completed 60 steps for the entire 1-minute test duration.

Anaerobic Capacity (kgm · min^{-1}) = 80 × [(0.40 × 60)/1] × 1.33

= [80 × (24/1)] ×1.33

= 80 × 24.0 × 1.33

= 2553 (kgm · min^{-1})

Conversion to Watts (6.12 kgm · min^{-1} = 1 W)

Watts = 2553 ÷ 6.12

= 417 W

Classification for Anaerobic Capacity		
	Male Power (W)	**Female Power (W)**
Athlete	>500	>320
Above Average	≥400	≥295
Average	360 - 399	240 - 295
Below Average	<360	<240

Activity 2 **Yo-Yo Intermittent Recovery Level 1 Test**

Activity Description

The interaction between energy systems is tested with increasing intensities and durations of training. It is well known that repeat anaerobic exercise and intermittent sport-based activities benefit from higher levels of cardiorespiratory fitness. This is due to reduced metabolic disruption during the activity as well as a more rapid ability to recover. The Yo-Yo Intermittent Recovery Level 1 Test provides useful data as to the level of cardiorespiratory fitness and buffering capacity of the body. The test involves running between two markers 20 meters apart at select running speeds, followed by an active break of 10 seconds before running 40 meters again. At regular intervals, the required running speed increases. The test continues until the participant can no longer keep up with the required pace. Even though it is a sprint-based test, it has demonstrated greater sensitivity in measuring performance changes than maximum oxygen uptake (VO_2max). Furthermore, since sub-maximal test performance and heart rates have been observed, non-exhaustive versions of this test can be used during competitive periods with young/elderly subjects as well as athletes recovering from injury.

Equipment

- Flat and non-slip surface (minimum length of 40 meters)
- Measuring tape (>30 meters)
- Stop watch
- Cones
- YYIR1 test audio and speaker
- Performance recording sheet

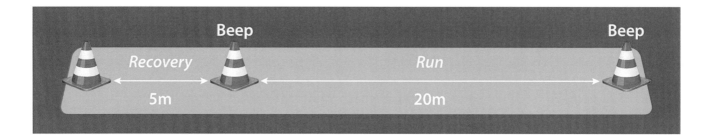

Procedures

Step 1 Measure and set up the cones for the assessment. Make sure the subject is familiar with the test prior to implementation and include practice as part of the warm-up.

Step 2 **Start Test:** On the initial beep, the subject runs 20m from the first to the second cone. A second beep will sound as the subject reaches the second cone to indicate the half way mark (assists with pacing). The subject must then run back 20m reaching the cone prior to the subsequent beep.

Step 3 The first shuttle is set to a cadence of 10 km/hour. The cadence is then increased within incremental stages as presented in the following example.

Step 4 The test is terminated when the client fails to finish 2 consecutive shuttles before the second beep sounds.

Step 5 VO_2max is obtained using the formula: **VO_2max = IR distance (m) $\times$ 0.0084 + 36.4**

Shuttle #	Speed Stage	Speed Level	Speed (km/hr)	Accumulated Distance (m)
1	1	5	10.0	40
2	2	8	12.0	80
3	3	11	13.0	120
4	3	11	13.0	160
5	4	12	13.5	200
6	4	12	13.5	240
7	4	12	13.5	280
8	5	13	14.0	320
9	5	13	14.0	360
10	5	13	14.0	400
11	5	13	14.0	440
12	6	14	14.5	480
13	6	14	14.5	520
14	6	14	14.5	560
15	6	14	14.5	600
16	6	14	14.5	640
17	6	14	14.5	680
18	6	14	14.5	720
19	6	14	14.5	760

Scoring System

Step 6   The test is comprised of up to 91 shuttles and can last up to approximately 29 minutes; however, it usually only takes between 6-20 minutes for level 1. Scores can be presented in three ways: 1) total distance (meters); 2) level achieved; or 3) VO_2max. The results normally report the speed attained plus number of shuttles, but many reference the VO_2 prediction instead of performing submaximal VO_2 tests to track changes in conditioning. Record each.

Distance achieved _____   Level Achieved _____   Speed attained _____ VO_2max _____

Yo-Yo Intermittent Recovery Test - Level 1

Speed Level	Shuttle No.	Speed (km/hr)	Level Time (s)	Accumulated Shuttle Dist (m)	Cumulative Time* (s)	Approx VO₂max (ml/min/kg)	Speed Level	Shuttle No.	Speed (km/hr)	Level Time (s)	Accumulated Shuttle Dist (m)	Cumulative Time* (s)	Approx VO₂max (ml/min/kg)
5	1	10	14.4	40	00:24	36.74	18	4	16.5	8.7	1880	15:29	52.19
9	1	12	12.5	80	00:46	37.07	18	5	16.5	8.7	1920	15:48	52.53
11	1	13	11.1	120	01:07	37.41	18	6	16.5	8.7	1960	16:07	52.86
11	2	13	11.1	160	01:29	37.74	18	7	16.5	8.7	2000	16:25	53.20
12	1	13.5	10.7	200	01:49	38.08	18	8	16.5	8.7	2040	16:44	53.54
12	2	13.5	10.7	240	02:10	38.42	19	1	17	8.5	2080	17:03	53.87
12	3	13.5	10.7	280	02:31	38.75	19	2	17	8.5	2120	17:21	54.21
13	1	14	10.3	320	02:51	39.09	19	3	17	8.5	2160	17:39	54.54
13	2	14	10.3	360	03:11	39.42	19	4	17	8.5	2200	17:58	54.88
13	3	14	10.3	400	03:31	39.76	19	5	17	8.5	2240	18:16	55.22
13	4	14	10.3	440	03:52	40.10	19	6	17	8.5	2280	18:35	55.55
14	1	14.5	9.9	480	04:12	40.43	19	7	17	8.5	2320	18:53	55.89
14	2	14.5	9.9	520	04:32	40.77	19	8	17	8.5	2360	19:12	56.22
14	3	14.5	9.9	560	04:51	41.10	20	1	17.5	8.2	2400	19:30	56.56
14	4	14.5	9.9	600	05:11	41.44	20	2	17.5	8.2	2440	19:48	56.90
14	5	14.5	9.9	640	05:31	41.78	20	3	17.5	8.2	2480	20:07	57.23
14	6	14.5	9.9	680	05:51	42.11	20	4	17.5	8.2	2520	20:25	57.57
14	7	14.5	9.9	720	06:11	42.45	20	5	17.5	8.2	2560	20:43	57.90
14	8	14.5	9.9	760	06:31	42.78	20	6	17.5	8.2	2600	21:01	58.24
15	1	15	9.6	800	06:51	43.12	20	7	17.5	8.2	2640	21:19	58.58
15	2	15	9.6	840	07:10	43.46	20	8	17.5	8.2	2680	21:38	58.91
15	3	15	9.6	880	07:30	43.79	21	1	18	8.0	2720	21:56	59.25
15	4	15	9.6	920	07:50	44.13	21	2	18	8.0	2760	22:14	59.58
15	5	15	9.6	960	08:09	44.46	21	3	18	8.0	2800	22:32	59.92
15	6	15	9.6	1000	08:29	44.80	21	4	18	8.0	2840	22:50	60.26
15	7	15	9.6	1040	08:48	45.14	21	5	18	8.0	2880	23:08	60.59
15	8	15	9.6	1080	09:08	45.47	21	6	18	8.0	2920	23:26	60.93
16	1	15.5	9.3	1120	09:27	45.81	21	7	18	8.0	2960	23:44	61.26
16	2	15.5	9.3	1160	09:47	46.14	21	8	18	8.0	3000	24:02	61.60
16	3	15.5	9.3	1200	10:06	46.48	22	1	18.5	7.8	3040	24:19	61.94
16	4	15.5	9.3	1240	10:25	46.82	22	2	18.5	7.8	3080	24:37	62.27
16	5	15.5	9.3	1280	10:44	47.15	22	3	18.5	7.8	3120	24:55	62.61
16	6	15.5	9.3	1320	11:04	47.49	22	4	18.5	7.8	3160	25:13	62.94
16	7	15.5	9.3	1360	11:23	47.82	22	5	18.5	7.8	3200	25:31	63.28
16	8	15.5	9.3	1400	11:42	48.16	22	6	18.5	7.8	3240	25:48	63.62
17	1	16	9	1440	12 01	48.50	22	7	18.5	7.8	3280	26:06	63.95
17	2	16	9	1480	12:20	48.83	22	8	18.5	7.8	3320	26:24	64.29
17	3	16	9	1520	12:39	49.17	23	1	19	7.6	3360	26:42	64.62
17	4	16	9	1560	12:58	49.50	23	2	19	7.6	3400	26:59	64.96
17	5	16	9	1600	13:17	49.84	23	3	19	7.6	3440	27:17	65.30
17	6	16	9	1640	13:36	50.18	23	4	19	7.6	3480	27:34	65.63
17	7	16	9	1680	13:55	50.51	23	5	19	7.6	3520	27:52	65.97
17	8	16	9	1720	14:14	50.85	23	6	19	7.6	3560	28:09	66.30
18	1	16.5	8.7	1760	14:33	51.18	23	7	19	7.6	3600	28:27	66.64
18	2	16.5	8.7	1800	14:52	51.52	23	8	19	7.6	3640	28:45	66.98
18	3	16.5	8.7	1840	15:10	51.86							

*Cumulative time includes 10 second recovery period between shuttles

Human Physiology Applications

Activity 3 Assessment of Resting Heart Rate

Activity Description

Exercise professionals are often required to assess a client's heart rate via manual palpation. Palpation simply refers to using the sense of touch to monitor or assess a physiological variable or structure of the body. The common carotid artery sites are located on both sides of the frontal aspect of the neck. Each is found in the groove formed by the larynx and the sternocleido-mastoid muscles just below the mandible. The carotid pulse is taken by placing the first two fingers of the hand in the groove and gently pressing inward. You will feel the pulse immediately if the location site is correct. There has been some evidence to suggest that the pressure exerted from the palpation of this site may cause the baroreceptors in the carotid sinus to cause a temporary decreased heart rate response in some individuals. For this reason, it is recommended to wait a few seconds when assessing the pulse before starting the count. Additionally, caution should be taken not to press too hard against the artery as the possibility of fainting or lightheadedness may result. This is of most concern during a post-exercise assessment.

Palpation of the radial artery is performed by placing the first two fingers near the distal end of the radius, just below the base of the thumb. This is the location where the normally deep-running radial artery travels superficially into the hand. By placing the first two fingers over this region and gently pressing, the radial pulse can be palpated. There may be some difficulty locating this pulse in individuals who have large amounts of subcutaneous fat, a weak pulse, or deep-lying vessels. In cases such as these, the carotid pulse may better serve as the palpation site. The thumb should **not** be used to palpate a subject's pulse because it has a pulse of its own which may interfere with proper palpation of the site.

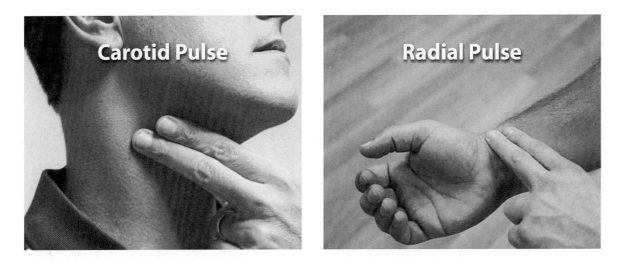

The length of time a pulse is taken is dependent on the purpose of the measurement and the accuracy required. A pulse count that is taken for only 10 seconds may have a larger degree of error than one that is taken for 30 seconds or a full minute due to possible tester error and pulse deviations. For accurate resting pulse counts, the NCSF recommends taking the measurement for a full 60 seconds to determine the subject's resting heart rate in beats/min. During exercise, smaller time increments are used to assess the subject's heart rate, usually 10 or 15 second counts.

Procedures

Using the guidelines below, administer a resting heart rate assessment on a volunteer.

Step 1 Administration of any resting physiological parameter requires the subject to be in a relaxed seated position with both feet flat on the floor. He or she should refrain from any activity for a minimum of 10 minutes prior to measuring the resting heart rate. This will ensure that the heart rate is at a true resting state.

Step 2 Ask the subject if they have consumed any stimulants such as caffeine or nicotine, or if they have taken any medications prior to the evaluation, as this may affect resting values.

Step 3 Following the aforementioned palpation protocols, administer a 30-second and 60-second resting heart rate assessment using both the radial and carotid palpation sites. As you palpate your lab partner's pulse, they should palpate his or her own pulse using the other palpation site. This may aid in accuracy and increase experience at palpating different sites. At the conclusion of the predetermined evaluation period the tester and subject should compare values to ensure that the tester and subject are accurately monitoring the correct pulse count.

Step 4 Record the heart rate values in the spaces provided and compare your results to the norms for resting heart rate.

30-second pulse count

_____ beats × 2 = _____ beats/min

60-second pulse count

_____ beats/min

	MEN					WOMEN				
%	20-29 y	30-39 y	40-49 y	50-59 y	60+ y	20-29 y	30-39 y	40-49 y	50-59 y	60+ y
90	50	50	50	50	52	55	55	55	55	52
80	54	55	54	55	55	59	58	60	60	57
70	58	58	58	58	58	60	62	62	61	60
60	60	60	60	60	60	63	65	64	64	62
50	63	63	62	63	62	65	68	66	67	64
40	66	65	65	65	65	70	70	70	69	66
30	70	68	69	68	68	72	74	72	72	72
20	72	72	72	72	72	75	76	76	75	74
10	80	77	78	77	77	84	82	80	83	79

Resting Heart Rate in Men and Women (beats/min)

Activity 4 Assessment of Resting Blood Pressure

Activity Description

Blood pressure (BP) is a product of cardiac output (heart rate x stroke volume) and total peripheral resistance, which is measured in millimeters of mercury (mmHg). The administration of a blood pressure evaluation prior to beginning an exercise program will assist the fitness professional in making activity decisions for the client; identify a possible hypertensive condition requiring medical referral; establish a baseline value to which future assessment comparisons can be made; and provide the client with valuable information pertaining to health status.

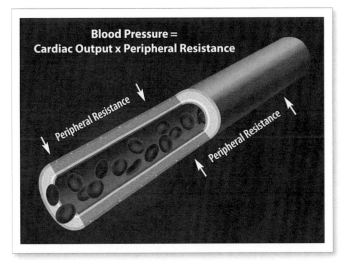

There are several non-invasive tools available to assess and monitor a client's blood pressure. This includes the use of a sphygmomanometer (pronounced sfig-mo-ma-nom-e-ter), commonly referred to as a manometer. Manometers are available in several types, from mercury or needle gauge to electronic measuring instruments. These devices measure the blood pressure in mmHg. This lab will present general guidelines for the administration of a resting blood pressure assessment using an electronic cuff manometer. Individual administration protocols are determined by the device used (digital, mercury, aneroid, etc.) It is recommended that you become proficient using several types of manometers as future work environments may have different measuring devices or protocol requirements. It is also important to note that if an individual's first assessment is elevated above acceptable guidelines or previously-established values, one should repeat the assessment again after a few minutes. The "white coat syndrome" may adversely affect readings and/or the subject may need more time to relax in a comfortable seated position.

Equipment

- Electronic/digital BP cuff
- Tape measure

Procedures

Step 1 Select Cuff Size: There are several cuff sizes available for manometers. Measure the resting arm circumference of your subject using a metric measuring tape. The following chart will assist you in identifying the correct cuff size for the evaluation (1 inch = 2.54 cm). An improper fitting cuff may provide the user with false information. Using a cuff that is too small may overestimate blood pressure, whereas cuffs that are too large may underestimate blood pressure.

Upper Arm Circumference (cm)	Type of Cuff	Bladder Size (cm)
33-47	Large Adult	42 x 15
25-35	Adult	24 x 12.5
18-26	Child	21.5 x 10

Step 2   Subject Preparation: Certain preparation procedures should be followed prior to the administration of any resting physiological assessment. In addition to the normal preparation instruction for the administration of resting heart rate assessment, it is extremely important to give your subject at least five minutes to relax in a comfortable environment prior to the blood pressure measurement or re-measurement. Sleeveless shirts, blouses, or loose-fitting sleeves are recommended as the cuff should be in contact with the skin to increase testing accuracy. If the sleeve appears to fit tightly around the subject's arm when rolled up, the shirt should be removed. This will ensure that the artery is not further occluded, which will skew results. The subject should also be in a seated position when the cuff is placed over the arm. This will automatically place the subject's antecubital space at heart level.

Step 3   Cuff Placement: There has been much debate over which arm to monitor when assessing the blood pressure of an individual. Researchers recommend that the right arm be used for the assessment. This is partly because of the remote possibility that the genetic anomaly of coarctation between the aorta and subclavian artery will cause an elevated blood pressure, and if the pressure is within normal ranges here, it is likely to be normal everywhere.

When placing the cuff over the arm the tester should look for the arterial reference indicator located near the center of the cuff. This should be positioned over the brachial artery. The lower edge of the cuff should be about 1 inch above the antecubital space, which is located on the frontal aspect of the elbow. The brachial artery travels through a groove formed by the bifurcation of the triceps and biceps brachii. If you are using a manual manometer and stethoscope you should locate the artery by palpating the area with the first 2 fingers at the medial antecubital space. This is the location for the head of the stethoscope.

Electronic Manometer

Step 4   Inflating/Deflating the Cuff: The determination of blood pressure using the typical manometer device is based upon the sounds made by vibrations from the vascular walls. These sounds are referred to as Korotkoff sounds (named after their discoverer in 1905). When the cuff is inflated to a predetermined level (see below) the flow of blood through the artery becomes streamlined and the blood begins to "back up" behind the obstruction (in the case of blood pressure reading this will take place on the proximal end of the cuff). As the pressure is released there is a bolus of blood escaping the obstruction and moving through the artery. This bolus causes vascular vibrations that result in a faint sound (systolic pressure reading). As the cuff continues to release the air from the bladder more blood escapes through the obstruction caused by the inflated cuff, which causes an even greater vibration and louder sounds picked up by the sensors. As the pressure is further released from the cuff the blood eventually ceases to vibrate during ventricular contraction. This is due to the lack of obstruction from the decreased pressure placed on the artery from the cuff. The point of the "disappearance of sound" is the diastolic pressure.

Cuff Inflation Pressure(s)

- 165 mmHg females

- 185 mmHg males

- 20 mmHg above expected or known systolic blood pressure

- 30 mmHg above the disappearance of the radial pulse

Be sure to follow the manufacturer's directions when using automated devices as administration protocols may vary slightly. **Note:** Place the cuff on the subject and position it in the correct location before turning on an electronic device and inflating. The sensors of the cuff will often detect movement and may not provide accurate results if this step is not performed.

Step 5 **Record Results:** Record all results in the spaces provided below. The results will be used to clear a subject for entrance into an exercise program and used for future comparisons.

BP 1 _____/_____ mmHg   **BP 2** _____/_____ mmHg

Blood Pressure Category	SYSTOLIC mm Hg (Upper Number)		DIASTOLIC mm Hg (Lower Number)
NORMAL	Less than 120	and	Less than 80
ELEVATED	120 - 129	and	Less than 80
HIGH BLOOD PRESSURE (Hypertension) Stage 1	130 - 139	or	80 - 89
HIGH BLOOD PRESSURE (Hypertension) Stage 2	140 or Higher	or	90 or Higher
HYPERTENSIVE CRISIS Consult Your Doctor Immediately	Higher than 180	and/or	Higher than 120

Human Physiology Applications Quiz

1. The anaerobic power step test requires primary support from which energy systems?

   _____ a. Phosphagen and aerobic
   _____ b. Glycolytic and aerobic
   _____ c. Phosphagen and glycolytic
   _____ d. None of the above are correct

2. What is the duration of the anaerobic power step test?

   _____ a. 30 seconds
   _____ b. 60 seconds
   _____ c. 90 seconds
   _____ d. 120 seconds

3. Which of the following is not correct concerning the anaerobic power step test?

   _____ a. A 16-inch box is used for clients of all sizes
   _____ b. A step is not counted if the client's hip remains flexed or the leg is not fully straightened
   _____ c. Classification for anaerobic capacity is provided in Watts
   _____ d. The average of the two 60-second efforts is taken for classifying anaerobic power

4. The first shuttle of the Yo-Yo intermittent recovery test starts at:

   _____ a. 10 km/hour
   _____ b. 12 km/hour
   _____ c. 14 km/hour
   _____ d. Maximum speed

5. The Yo-Yo intermittent recovery test is terminated when:

   _____ a. The client needs a recovery period of 10 seconds between shuttles
   _____ b. The client fails to finish a shuttle within 5 seconds of the start of each beep
   _____ c. The client fails to finish two consecutive shuttles when the beep sounds
   _____ d. The client fails to decelerate before the recovery cone behind the starting point

6. Scores for the Yo-Yo intermittent recovery test can be presented as:

    ____ a. Total distance covered in meters
    ____ b. Speed level or stage achieved
    ____ c. A VO$_2$max value
    ____ d. All of the above are correct

7. Palpation of which of the following pulse sites can be associated with lightheadedness in certain situations?

    ____ a. Brachial artery
    ____ b. Pedal artery
    ____ c. Carotid artery
    ____ d. Radial artery

8. Which of the following is correct concerning a resting heart rate assessment?

    ____ a. The pulse should be taken using the thumb for the broadest surface coverage
    ____ b. The pulse should be taken while the client is standing motionless for 15 seconds
    ____ c. A pulse assessment taken for 10 seconds may have a larger degree of error than a 30-second assessment
    ____ d. The radial pulse is generally stronger than the carotid among obese clients

9. If assessing the resting blood pressure of an adult male, the cuff should be inflated to at least:

    ____ a. 155 mmHg
    ____ b. 170 mmHg
    ____ c. 185 mmHg
    ____ d. 220 mmHg

10. What systolic measure is considered stage 1 hypertension?

    ____ a. 110 mmHg
    ____ b. 120 mmHg
    ____ c. 130 mmHg
    ____ d. 140 mmHg

Human Physiology Applications

◆ Health Appraisal & Screening

This lab corresponds to the following text – Chapter 4: Pages 167-170; Chapter 5: Pages 208-220; Chapter 6: Pages 240-249; Chapter 7: Page 269

Activity 1 **Informed Consent**

Activity Description

Prior to a person engaging in physical activity under the supervision of an exercise professional, there are several "clearance" procedures that should be performed to reduce the risk of liability in the event of a training accident or incident. Professional screening practices reduce professional liability, fosters communication with regard to the benefits and risks of physical activity, and eases client concern for exercise safety. The first of these procedures is the administration of an Informed Consent Form. The form serves several functions in the initial education of a client as to what to expect with exercise participation.

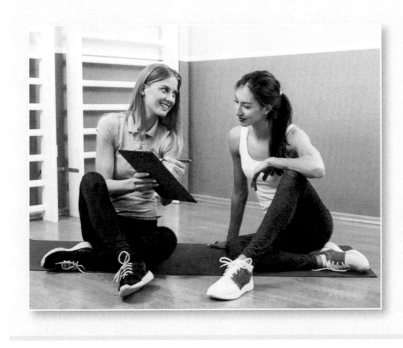

Benefits of Client Screening

1. Educating the client about relative health risks associated with their lifestyle, behaviors, and history.

2. Identifying current health status compared to recommended ranges.

3. Providing data that will be used to create a needs analysis as the basis for the exercise prescription.

4. Establishing starting points and predictions of performance.

5. Identifying particular interests, aptitudes, or possible limitations.

Exercise, as with all other forms of physical exertion, has some degree of risk. Although the risks for participation in an exercise program or testing protocol are relatively low, and whilst most health professionals believe the benefits outweigh the risks, it is important to ensure an optimal benefit-to-risk ratio when making activity decisions. Additionally, a client should know the assumed risks of participation. This requires that the risks are thoroughly explained to the client before they engage in any mode of physical activity.

From a legal standpoint, any participant involved in physical activity for which another party is responsible for the structure, prescription, organization, or assessment of the participant's actions must give informed consent for the activity to be legally defensible. Informed consent is intended to show that the participant entered into the activity or testing procedure with full knowledge of the procedures, relative risks, expected physiological occurrence, benefits, and alternatives, if applicable. To give valid consent, an individual must be of legal age and have all mental faculties. They must fully understand the importance and relevance of the material risks and provide a voluntary consent, preferably in writing, for increased legal protection. Written consent holds greater merit should questions to the procedure arise on a later occasion.

One of the fallacies regarding informed consent is that it relinquishes any and all responsibility in the event of a training accident. This is not necessarily the case. Nothing will protect the exercise professional against liability stemming from professional negligence (failing to explain and have the client sign, a well written consent form is the first "negligent" thing a trainer can do). However, if an informed consent is signed by the client which states the activities to be performed and the risks involved, the exercise professional can better protect themselves in the event of an incident. Additionally, the client accepts a level of accountability once they are made aware of the risks associated with the activities; which in the case of informed consent, occurs before they are undertaken. This allows a client to make an educated and willful decision to participate.

Legal action arising from the informed consent procedure frequently occurs when the injured party claims negligence based on the explanation or administration of the Informed Consent. The result of the suit is often based on the informed consent process and the conduct by which the professional implemented the test or activity. This means that the informed consent must be as detailed as possible with regard to the exercises, assessments, and training procedures used – including modes, intensities, and possible health risks (in some cases death). From a communication standpoint, exercise professionals should explain the document and identify to the client that there are risks associated with the activity procedures and describe measures to address specific concerns arising from activity participation. This will create an open trainer/client relationship and assist in the education process for the client.

Procedures

Step 1 *Purpose and explanation of the procedure.* Thoroughly explain all the activities the subject will be participating in, as well as the rationale behind the activity selection.

Step 2 *Explanation of risks.* Identify possible risks involved with basic exercise and the activities for which they will be participating.

Step 3 *Explanation of benefits.* Explain the specific positive role the activity will play in promoting their health/fitness.

Step 4 *Procedures of the test or activity.* Provide clear instructions and timetables related to any activity so the subject knows exactly what to expect and has a good idea of what they will be doing.

Step 5 *Physiological expectations from the physical effort.* Identify the normal physical occurrences the subject may experience during the activity.

Step 6 *Explain confidentiality.* Identify that all information gathered during the test or activity is confidential.

Step 7 *Inquiries and freedom from consent.* Answer any questions the subject may have with regard to the activity and clearly state that they have the option to refuse or stop participation at any time.

Step 8 *Emergency contact information.* Although this is also provided on the Health Status Questionnaire (HSQ), it is beneficial to have this information in a readily-accessible area.

INFORMED CONSENT

Purpose and Explanation of Service

I understand that the purpose of the exercise program is to develop and maintain healthy levels of cardiorespiratory fitness, body composition, flexibility, muscular strength and endurance. A specific exercise plan will be given to me, based on my needs and abilities. All exercise prescription components will comply with known, proper, exercise program protocols. The program includes, but is not limited to, aerobic exercise, flexibility training, and strength training. All programming is designed to place a gradually increasing workload on the body in order to improve overall fitness.

Risks

I understand, and have been informed, that there exists the possibility of adverse changes when engaging in a physical activity program. I have been informed that these changes could include abnormal blood pressure, fainting, disorders of heart rhythm, stroke and very rare instances of heart attack or even death. I have been told that every effort will be made to minimize these occurrences by proper screening and by precautions and observations taken during the exercise session. I understand that there is a risk of injury, heart attack, or even death as a result of my participation in an exercise program, but knowing those risks, it is my desire to partake in the recommended activities.

Benefits

I understand that participation in an exercise program has many health-related benefits. These may include improvements in body composition, range of motion, musculoskeletal strength and endurance, and cardiorespiratory efficiency. Furthermore, regular exercise can improve blood pressure and lipid profile, metabolic function, and decreases the risk of cardiovascular disease.

Physiological Experience

I have been informed that during my participation in the exercise program I will be asked to complete physical activities that may elicit physiological responses/symptoms that include, but are not limited to, the following: elevated heart rate, elevated blood pressure, sweating, fatigue, increased respiration, muscle soreness, cramping, and nausea.

Confidentiality and Use of Information

I have been informed that the information obtained in this exercise program will be treated as privileged and confidential and will not be released or revealed to any person without my express written consent. Any other information obtained, however, will be used only by the program staff to evaluate my exercise status as needed.

Inquiries and Freedom of Consent

I have been given an opportunity to ask questions about the exercise program. I further understand that there are also other remote health risks. Despite the fact that a complete accounting of all these remote risks has not been provided to me, I still desire to proceed with the exercise program. I acknowledge that I have read this document in its entirety or that it has been read to me if I have been unable to read same. I consent to the rendition of all services and procedures as explained herein by all program personnel.

_____
Date

_____
Participant's Signature

_____
Witness's Signature

_____
Exercise Professional Signature

Activity 2 **Health Status Questionnaire**

Activity Description

The second step in the screening process is to employ the use of health appraisal tools prior to client engagement in physical activity. Administering a health appraisal to a new client prior to his or her participation in physical activity (exercise testing and any other form of physical activity) will:

1 Provide the exercise professional with information relevant to the safety of fitness testing before beginning exercise training

2 Identify any known diseases and related risk factors as well as potentially-preventable chronic conditions

3 Identify additional factors that require special consideration in the development of an appropriate program

4 Provide a platform to engage and educate clients

5 Provide insight into needed lifestyle interventions and exercise programming that will optimize adherence, minimize risks, and maximize benefits

The Health Status Questionnaire (HSQ) is a widely-used health appraisal tool for clearing participants into an exercise program. It is a four-part screening tool designed to provide the fitness professional with information about: any diagnosed medical problems, characteristics that increase the risk of health problems, signs or symptoms that increase the risk of health problems, and lifestyle behaviors related to positive or negative health. The HSQ is one of the first tools a personal trainer will employ prior to a client engaging in any form of physical activity under their supervision. The information provided on the HSQ can help to reduce trainer liability and is very beneficial in the creation of a comprehensive health profile of the prospective new client. The health profile is used to not only document and assess risk stratification, but also to help educate the client as to potential health problems stemming from lifestyle decisions, predisposed hereditary issues, and/or current medical conditions that can be positively affected by exercise.

The document is intended to be administered as an oral questionnaire. The rationale behind this method of implementation is to use the questions as probes for more information and greater detail about certain answers. ***Then, depending on the responses to the questions on the HSQ, the subject can be referred for medical clearance, if indicated, and/or placed into one of three categories; to 1) a medically-supervised program, 2) an exercise professional supervised program or 3) cleared for unrestricted activity.*** There are also specific action codes associated with many of the questions/responses to help the fitness professional choose a correct course of action when, and if, special procedures are necessary prior to beginning an exercise program. Knowing the correct course of action with regard to an individual's personal screening information is a vital aspect of the exercise professional's job description.

Procedures

The following case study includes a completed HSQ document. Review the document and identify any responses related to the following: diagnosed medical problems, characteristics that increase the risk of health problems, signs or symptoms indicative of health problems, and lifestyle behaviors related to positive or negative health. You should also identify items that may positively or negatively affect the sample client's health and/or exercise program adherence.

Step 1 Review the HSQ document and identify significant and relevant findings.

Step 2 Stratify the risk by listing the findings in order of relevance and document the action codes for each.

Step 3 Analyze the findings and make a program participation decision for the sample subject.

Program participation recommendation: _____

_____

HEALTH STATUS QUESTIONNAIRE

SECTION ONE – *GENERAL INFORMATION*

1. Date: _7/6/2018_

2. Name: _John Delaney_

3. Mailing Address: _15 Elm St. Merribel, PA 18623_   Phone (C): _555-347-2830_

        Phone (W): _____

   Email: _JMoney@2times.com_

4. *EI* Personal Physician: _Dr. Andrew Vincent_   Phone: _____

   Physician Address: _____   Fax: _____

5. *EI* Person to contact in case of Emergency: _Mary Delaney_   Phone: _Same_

6. Gender (circle one):   Female   (*RF* Male)

7. *RF* Date of Birth: _06/23/68_

8. Height: _5' 10"_   Weight: _205_

9. Number of hours worked per week: Less than 20   20-40   (41-50)   over 50

10. *SLA* More than 25% of the time at your job is spent *(circle all that apply)*:

    (Sitting at desk)   Lifting loads   Standing   Walking   Driving

SECTION TWO – *CURRENT MEDICAL INFORMATION*

11. Date of last medical physical exam: _06/14/2018_

12. Circle all medicine taken or prescribed within the last 6 months:

Blood thinner *MC*	Epilepsy medication *SEP*	Nitroglycerin *MC*
Diabetic *MC*	Heart rhythm medication *MC*	Other: _____
Digitalis *MC*	(High blood pressure medication *MC*)	
Diuretic *MC*	Insulin *MC*	

13. Please list any orthopedic conditions. Include any injuries in the last six months.

    ACL tear in High School – Surgically repaired 1986

14. Any of these health symptoms that occur frequently *(two or more times/month)* require medical attention.

    Please check any that apply.

    a. ___ Cough up blood *MC*   g. ___ Swollen joints *MC*

    b. ___ Abdominal pain *MC*   h. ___ Feel faint *MC*

    c. ___ Low-back pain *MC*   i. ___ Dizziness *MC*

    d. ___ Leg pain *MC*   j. ___ Breathlessness with slight exertion *MC*

    e. ___ Arm or shoulder pain *MC*   k. ___ Palpitation or fast heart beat *MC*

    f. ___ Chest pain RF *MC*   l. ___ Unusual fatigue with normal activity *MC*

    Other: _____

HEALTH STATUS QUESTIONNAIRE

SECTION THREE – *MEDICAL HISTORY*

15. Please circle any of the following for which you have been diagnosed or treated by a physician or health professional:

Alcoholism *SEP*	Diabetes *SEP*	Kidney problem *MC*
Anemia, sickle cell *SEP*	Emphysema *SEP*	Mental illness *SEP*
Anemia, other *SEP*	Epilepsy *SEP*	Neck strain *SLA*
Asthma *SEP*	Eye problems *SLA*	Obesity *RF*
Back strain *SLA*	Gout *SLA*	Phlebitis *MC*
Bleeding trait *SEP*	Hearing loss *SLA*	Rheumatoid arthritis *SLA*
Bronchitis, chronic *SEP*	Heart problems *MC*	Stress *RF*
Stroke *MC*	Cancer *SEP*	(High blood pressure *SLA*)
Thyroid problem *SEP*	Cirrhosis *MC*	HIV *SEP*
Ulcer *SEP*	Concussion *MC*	Hypoglycemia *SEP*
Congenital defect *SEP*	Hyperlipidemia *RF*	Other: _____

16. Circle any operations that you have had:

Back *SLA*	Heart *MC*	Kidneys *SLA*	Eyes *SLA*	(Joints *SLA*)	Neck *SLA*
Ears *SLA*	Hernia *SLA*	Lungs *SLA*	Other: _____		

17. *RF* Circle any of the following who died of heart attack before age 55:

Father   Brother   Son

18. *RF* Circle any of the following who died of heart attack before age 65:

Mother   Sister   Daughter

SECTION FOUR – *HEALTH-RELATED BEHAVIORS*

19. Have you ever smoked?   Yes   (No)
20. *RF* Do you currently smoke?   Yes   (No)
21. *RF* If you are a smoker, indicate the number smoked per day:

Cigarettes: 40 or more   20-39   10-19   1-9

Cigars or pipes only: 5 or more or any inhaled less than 5

22. *RF* Do you exercise regularly?   Yes   (No)
23. Last physical fitness test: ____High School____
24. How many days a week do you accumulate 30 minutes of moderate activity?

(0)   1   2   3   4   5   6   7

25. How many days per week do you normally spend at least 20 minutes in vigorous exercise?

(0)   1   2   3   4   5   6   7

26. What activities do you engage in a least once per week? __Golf__
27. Weight now: __205 lbs.__   One year ago: __200 lbs.__   Age 21: __170 lbs.__

HEALTH STATUS QUESTIONNAIRE

SECTION FIVE – *HEALTH-RELATED ATTITUDES*

28. These are traits that have been associated with coronary-prone behavior. *Circle the number that corresponds to how you feel toward the following statement:*

I am an impatient, time-conscious, hard-driving individual.

(6) = Strongly agree   3 = Slightly disagree

5   = Moderately agree   2 = Moderately disagree

4   = Slightly agree   1 = Strongly disagree

29. How often do you experience "negative" stress from each of the following?

	RF Always	*RF* Usually	*RF* Frequently	Rarely	Never
Work:	___	___	X	___	___
Home or family:	___	___	___	X	___
Financial pressure:	___	___	___	X	___
Social pressure:	___	___	___	X	___
Personal health:	___	___	___	X	___

30. List everything not included on this questionnaire that may cause you problems in a fitness test or fitness program.

_____

_____

_____

_____

_____

_____

_____

_____

Action Codes

EI   = Emergency Information - must be readily available.

MC   = Medical Clearance needed - do not allow exercise without physician's permission.

SEP   = Special Emergency Procedures needed - do not let participant exercise alone; make sure the person's exercise partner knows what to do in case of an emergency.

RF   = Risk Factor of CHD (educational materials and workshops needed).

SLA   = Special or Limited Activities may be needed - you may need to include or exclude specific exercises.

Other (not marked)   = Personal information that may be helpful for files or research.

Activity 3 **Health Behavior Questionnaire**

Activity Description

Identifying negative health behaviors and patterns is another important aspect of an exercise professional's role as a health provider. For optimal improvements in health and fitness to take place, the client must not only engage in regular sustained physical activity, but also change detrimental dietary and behavioral habits. Although the HSQ provides the personal trainer with important health related information, it is still incomplete with regard to the development of a complete client health profile. Many health-related behaviors correlate with the findings on the HSQ. The Health Behavior Questionnaire can be utilized by the personal trainer to better identify problem areas and assist with client behavior modification.

Procedures

Review the following sample behavior form that coincides with the sample subject in the previous HSQ case study. Analyze the responses, noting anything that may negatively affect the subject's overall health status or impede goal attainment. After reviewing the behavior form, reference the HSQ noting any current conditions that may be affected by his behavior patterns.

Step 1 *Explain confidentiality.* Inform subject that all information given will be kept private and confidential.

Step 2 *Importance of accurate completion.* Explain the purpose of the Health Behavior Questionnaire and the importance of answering all questions as accurately as possible as they will affect program decisions. No judgement is being placed upon the answers – denying facts or lying will make the exercise a waste of time.

Step 3 *Form administration.* Administer the Health Behavior Questionnaire to your subject by asking each question and recording the response.

Step 4 *Form review.* Review and evaluate the form to identify positive and negative behaviors that may affect current and future health status.

BEHAVIOR QUESTIONNAIRE

1. How many servings of fruits and vegetables do you eat per day?

   0   (1)   2   3+

2. How many servings of vegetables do you eat per day?

   0   (1)   2   3+

3. How many glasses (8 ounces) of water do you drink per day?

   0-3   (4-5)   6-7   8+

4. How many meals do you consume per day?

   1-2   (3-4)   5-6   7+

5. My fat consumption includes: *(circle all that apply)*

   Fatty fish (salmon, sardines)   (Butter)   Margarine   Olive oil   Safflower oil

   Peanut oil   (Corn oil)   (Mayonnaise)   (Cheese)   Whole milk   (Nuts)

BEHAVIOR QUESTIONNAIRE

6.   My bread/grain eating habit includes: *(circle all that apply)*
        (White bread)   Whole grain bread   (Dinner/breakfast rolls)
        (Regular crackers)   Whole grain crackers   Flavored crackers
        (White rice)   Brown rice   (Regular pasta)   Whole grain pasta

7. How often do you eat out?
        __X__ I eat out nearly every day
        ____ I eat out several times each week
        ____ I eat out a few times each month
        ____ I seldom or never eat out

8. My salty food habit is:
        ____ I rarely eat salty foods (chips, pickles, soups, added salt)
        __X__ Occasionally I eat salty foods
        ____ I regularly eat salty food
        ____ I add salt to the foods I eat

9.   My snacking habits include: *(circle all that apply)*
        Bagged chips   Candy bars   (Snack bars)   Protein bars
        Beef jerky   (Nuts)   Cheese sticks   Baked goods

10.   How often do you eat desert foods (cookies, cakes, sweets)?
        ____ I eat desert nearly every day
        ____ I eat desert several times each week
        __X__ I eat desert a few times each month
        ____ I seldom or never eat desert foods

11.   How often do you eat red or processed meat?
        ____ I eat red or processed meat nearly every day
        __X__ I eat red or processed meat several times each week
        ____ I eat red or processed meat a few times each month
        ____ I seldom or never eat red or processed meat

12.   How many alcoholic beverages do you consume per week?
                0-3   4-5   (6-7)   8+

13.   On average, I sleep ____ hours a night.
                3-4   (5-6)   7-8   8+

14.   What supplements do you take? *(circle all that apply)*
        (Multi-vitamin mineral)   Weight loss   Protein   Energy drink
        Other _____

15.   During the past 30 days, did you diet to lose weight or to keep from gaining weight?
                Yes   (No)
        If Yes, explain:_____

List positive and negative behaviors from the sample Behavior Questionnaire.

Behavior	Positive or Negative	Benefit or Consequence	Recommendation
Sample: Consumes red or processed meat regularly	*Negative*	*Increased risk for stomach and colon cancer*	*Decrease meat intake to recommended values 12-18 ounces week) – avoid processed meats*
Low fruit and vegetable intake			
Moderately-low water intake			
Mayonnaise consumption			
Bread/grain eating habits side with processed options			
Nut consumption			
Eats out nearly every day			

Behavior	Positive or Negative	Benefit or Consequence	Recommendation
Occasionally eats salty foods			
Snack bars			
Eats deserts only a few times a month			
Consumes 6-7 alcoholic beverages a week			
Sleeps only 5-6 hours per night			
Consumes a multi-vitamin/ mineral supplement			

Step 5 *Goal establishment.* Establish both short- and long-term behavior modification goals using the SMART system (Specific, Measurable, Achievable, Relevant and Time-bound).

Specific-Outcome	Measurement	Achievability Score	Goal Duration
Example: Increase sleep by 2 hours per night	Weekly average assessment	Moderate	1 month
Increase daily fruit, vegetable and whole grain intake			
Increase water intake			
Reduce processed grain, condiment, desert and meat intake			
Eat out only 1-2 times per week			
Cut out all foods that taste salty and minimize high-sodium products			
Cut alcohol intake down to 1-3 beverages per week (by half)			
Assess the need for taking a multi-vitamin/mineral supplement			

Step 6 *Review and evaluate.* Analyze the Health Behavior Questionnaire and identify connecting factors between the behaviors and the documented health concerns found on the HSQ document. Identify correlating factors from the HSQ and make recommendations.

Behavioral Issue	Correlating Factor	Recommendations to Achieve Goal
Sample: Inadequate sleep	Weight gain; increases stress levels	Keep a sleep log Set bed time alarm Record late-night popular show
High alcohol intake		
Low fruit, vegetable and whole grain intake		

Behavioral Issue	Correlating Factor	Recommendations to Achieve Goal
Moderately-low water intake		
Eats out almost every day		
Eats salty foods and processed meats		

Activity 4 **Needs Analysis**

Activity Description

The HSQ and the Health Behavior Questionnaire clearly provide more information than simply what is needed to make a program participation decision. Findings on the document can identify components of the exercise prescription based on the activities that meet the specific need of the risk factor or health problem. These findings can be further supported by a resting battery of tests to quantify the actual level of need. Diseases such as obesity, hypertension, and diabetes have defined protocols that best correct or manage the disease. When the HSQ identifies a problem, the protocols that provide the solution should be included in the exercise prescription.

Procedures

Using the following case study, identify the correct prescription components to meet the sample client's needs. Once the disease or health risk has been identified, complete the table by recommending a type of exercise or activity.

Step 1 Identify and list the disease or health risk associated with the measured score or value of the sample client.

Name: **Steve Murphy**

Sex: **Male**   Height: **6 ft**

Age: **57**   Weight: **220**

Evaluation Criteria	Score	Disease or Health Risk
Example: BMI	30	Obesity
Waist circumference	104 cm (41 inches)	
Systolic blood pressure	158 mmHg	
Diastolic blood pressure	112 mmHg	
Resting heart rate	75 beats/min	
Total cholesterol	289 mg/dl	
Fasting blood glucose	121 mg/dl	

Step 2   Using the list created from Step 1 identify the appropriate type of exercise (i.e. aerobic training) for each disease state or health risk. Then identify the mechanism of action by which improvements are experienced.

Disease or Health Risk	Type of Exercise	Mechanism of Action

Health Appraisal & Screening Quiz

1. Which of the following is the first screening document that should be implemented with a new client?

    ____ a. Health status questionnaire
    ____ b. Informed consent
    ____ c. Health behavior questionnaire
    ____ d. Needs analysis

2. True or False? An informed consent form must be implemented to protect the exercise professional from negligence.

    ____ a. True
    ____ b. False

3. Which of the following is not a section of an informed consent form?

    ____ a. Explanation of benefits
    ____ b. Explanation of risks
    ____ c. Explanation of adaptations to training
    ____ d. Explanation of confidentiality of information

4. The health status questionnaire can identify all of the following, except:

    ____ a. Genetic predisposition for specific performance improvements
    ____ b. Known diseases and related risk factors
    ____ c. Known physical limitations and special needs
    ____ d. Necessary lifestyle interventions for improved health

5. Which of the following screening forms is most useful for discerning lifestyle habits that are promoting health issues?

    ____ a. PARQ+
    ____ b. Informed consent
    ____ c. Physician release form
    ____ d. Health behavior questionnaire

6. Which of the following serves as a "to-do" list for the client, using information gleaned from the screening process to develop program activities?

_____ a. Informed consent
_____ b. Health status questionnaire
_____ c. Needs analysis
_____ d. PARQ+

7. Which of the following would be most beneficial for a client found to be hypertensive?

_____ a. Reduce plant-based fat intake
_____ b. Increase vitamin D intake
_____ c. Reduce sodium intake
_____ d. Increase fiber intake

8. Which of the following behaviors is associated with obesity?

_____ a. Frequent alcohol consumption
_____ b. Low fruit and vegetable intake
_____ c. High processed food intake
_____ d. All of the above

9. Which of the following would be the best choice for a client with prediabetes?

_____ a. Heavy strength training for neuromuscular system development
_____ b. Higher intensity circuit training
_____ c. Yoga
_____ d. Long-distance training in the fat-burning zone

10. Which of the following should be the primary focus for a client with cholesterol issues (e.g., hyperlipidemia)?

_____ a. Mobility training
_____ b. Power training
_____ c. Aerobic training
_____ d. Strength training

◆ Cardiorespiratory Fitness Testing

This lab corresponds to the following text - Chapter 7: Pages 306-311, 314-317

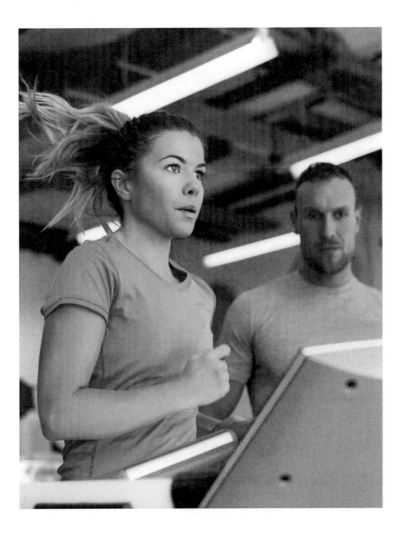

Activity 1 **Fitness Testing Preparation Checklist**

Activity Description

A key component to validity is subject pre-test preparation. Preparing the subject for the test requires specific directions on what to do or not to do prior to engaging in the activity. This means providing a detailed list to improve compliance with all test preparation protocols. A Fitness Testing Preparation Checklist is valuable for successful preparation and aids in improving validity of test results. The list attempts to identify factors that may change the results of the test from their true value. Personal trainers must be able to distinguish factors that have no effect on test scores from ones that may create false data.

Procedures

Complete the following Fitness Test Checklist using a volunteer subject. If any particular aspect of the checklist identifies a factor that may affect the lab outcome, document it and take the necessary steps to correct the situation prior to testing.

FITNESS TEST PREPARATION CHECKLIST

Subject Preparation

1. Subject has completed the informed consent. _____
2. Subject has been screened and cleared for participation. _____
3. Subject has read and understands the test procedures. _____
4. Subject understands the starting and stopping procedures. _____
5. Subject knows the stop test indicators. _____
6. Subject understands what is expected for each stage of the test. _____
7. Subject has complied with all pre-test instructions concerning:
    A. Rest _____
    B. Food _____
    C. Beverage and hydration status _____
    D. Drugs – including prescription, stimulants, depressants, alcohol, and tobacco _____
    E. Appropriate attire _____
8. Subject does not have illness or injury. _____
9. Subject is not fatigued, stressed, or anxious. _____
10. Subject is not on any medication (prescription or non-prescription). _____
11. Subject has participated in the proper warm-up procedure. _____

Tester Preparation

1. Test to be administered has been determined. _____
2. The protocols for administration are understood. _____
3. Equipment has been tested, calibrated, and is in good working order. _____
4. All necessary equipment, supplies, and recording sheets are ready. _____
5. The test environment is within acceptable limits for:
    A. Cleanliness _____
    B. Temperature _____
    C. Humidity _____
    D. Noise _____
6. The timing and sequence of testing are set. _____
7. The starting and stopping instructions are clear. _____
8. The subject has been prepared appropriately and meets all guidelines for testing. _____
9. The test atmosphere and environment are controlled. _____
10. Post test activities and responsibilities are set. _____
11. Emergency procedures are determined and understood. _____

Activity 2 **3 Minute Step Test**

Activity Description

One of the more common types of cardiorespiratory fitness field tests is the step test. In most cases, the tests last between 2-5 minutes, employing varying step-pace protocols. The tests are applicable for most apparently-healthy persons as they require limited movement economy and can be performed in almost any setting. The exercise intensity is generally low enough for most individuals to complete the prescribed duration, and high enough to sufficiently raise the heart rates of physically-fit clients to get an accurate assessment of their VO_2max. However, the test may be too intense for individuals with an extremely low fitness level, those that are obese, and for many individuals over the age of 65.

The physiological rationale for the prediction of maximal oxygen consumption is based upon the positive relationship between oxygen consumption and exercise. As with oxygen consumption, heart rate is linearly related to exercise. This means that heart rate and oxygen consumption are directly related. Although heart rates are not measured during the performance of the 3 Minute Step Test, there is enough evidence to support a high relationship between estimated exercise heart rates and the actual exercise heart rate.

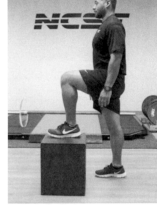

Equipment

- Metronome
- Stop watch
- 16.25-inch Step or Box
- Heart rate monitor (optional)

Procedures

The following activity requires you to administer the 3 Minute Step Test with a volunteer subject. Be sure to read through the entire lab prior to implementing this assessment.

Step 1 *Preparation.* Ensure that the subject:
   1. Has signed an informed consent form and has been cleared to participate in activity
   2. Has been checked for fitness preparation (Activity 1)

Step 2 *Stop Test Indicators.* Read and explain the following Stop Test Indicators to the subject.

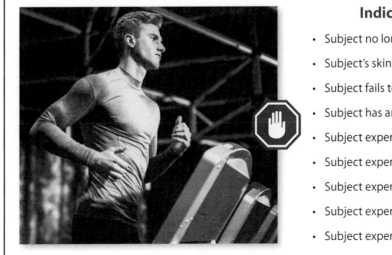

Indications for Test Termination

- Subject no longer feels comfortable doing the test.
- Subject's skin becomes pale.
- Subject fails to keep cadence for 20 seconds or more.
- Subject has an inability to focus attention.
- Subject experiences faintness, dizziness, or lightheadedness.
- Subject experiences upset stomach or vomiting symptoms.
- Subject experiences dysfunction in breathing.
- Subject experiences chest pain.
- Subject experiences side stitch, cramp, strain, fatigue.

Step 3 *Practice Stepping.* Skill acquisition is an important aspect to ensuring test validity and reliability. The subject must be comfortable and proficient at performing the assessment criterion, otherwise the test should not be performed until the movement skill is mastered, or another assessment protocol should be used in its place. The 3 Minute Step Test requires the use of a metronome set at 96 tones per minute for men and 88 tones per minute for women. For every tone, the subject must either step up or step down.

Once the metronome is operating at the designated tones per minute rate, have the subject face the step and instruct him or her to practice stepping up and down on the box or step using the following four-count cadence.

"Up-one"	Foot #1 goes to the top of the step
"Up-two"	The other foot (#2) follows to the top of the step
"Down-one"	Foot #1 descends to the floor
"Down-two"	Foot #2 descends to the floor

After the subject is able to successfully step up and down on the box or step at the correct cadence (usually about 30 seconds), have them sit for 2-3 minutes. This will allow the elevation in heart rate from the skill acquisition period to return to resting state.

Step 4 *Begin Assessment.* Start the metronome at the correct tone per minute cadence. Have the subject face the box and begin stepping whenever they feel comfortable. As soon as the subject takes the first step, the administrator should begin timing the assessment.

> *Clock time 0:00 – begin stepping*

Step 5 *Test Performance.* Have subject continue stepping on and off the box, staying in exact accordance with the cadence for the full 3 minutes of the test. The test administrator should visually assess the subject throughout the duration of the test for proper identification of any signs and symptoms that may require the test to be stopped (Step Test Indicators). The test administrator should also periodically ask the subject how they are feeling to assess the subject's relative rate of perceived exertion (RPE). The RPE for this type of sub-maximal assessment should not exceed 7 on a 1 to 10 scale or a 16 on a 1 to 20 scale.

> *Clock time 0:00 - 3:00 – step test administration*

Step 6 *Palpation Preparation.* When the stop watch reaches the three (3:00) minute mark have the subject stop stepping and sit down on the step. Be sure to keep the watch running as it will be used to assess the recovery heart rate of the subject. Locate the subject's radial pulse as the clock continues to run.

> *Clock time 3:00 – subject stops stepping and administrator palpates the radial pulse*

Step 7 *Recovery Heart Rate Palpation.* Once the stopwatch reads 3:05 the test administrator should begin counting the subject's recovery heart rate through the palpation of the radial artery. Monitoring of the subject's heart rate should start at the 3:05 mark and end at the 3:20 mark. This will provide the number of times the subject's heart has cycled in 15 seconds.

> *Clock time 3:05 - 3:20 – count pulse rate*

Step 8 Record the 15 second recovery heart rate and have subject perform a cool down.

> *Pulse rate for 15 seconds =_____*

Procedures for Estimating VO$_2$max

Step 1 *Calculate the estimated VO$_2$max.* To find the fitness score you will need the value from Step 8. Enter the subject's pulse rate into the following formula, this will provide the subject's predicted VO$_2$max (ml/kg/min).

Men: Estimated VO$_2$max = 111.33 − (0.42 × _____)

Women: Estimated VO$_2$max = 65.81 − (0.1847 × _____)

Enter score here _____ fitness score (ml/kg/min)

Step 2 *Calculate fitness level score.* Using the **Estimated VO$_2$max**, find the subject's fitness score using the table. The table includes the values for men and women, so it is important to refer to the correct gender values.

Enter score here _____

Sex	Age	Poor	Fair	Average	Good	Excellent
Men	<29	<25	25 - 33	34 - 42	43 - 52	53+
	30 - 39	<23	23 - 30	31 - 38	39 - 48	49+
	40 - 49	<20	20 - 26	27 - 35	36 - 44	45+
	50 - 59	<18	18 - 24	25 - 33	34 - 42	43+
	60 - 69	<16	16 - 22	23 - 30	31 - 40	41+
Women	<29	<24	24 - 30	31 - 37	38 - 48	49+
	30 - 39	<20	20 - 27	28 - 33	34 - 44	45+
	40 - 49	<17	17 - 23	24 - 30	31 - 41	42+
	50 - 59	<15	15 - 20	21 - 27	28 - 37	38+
	60 - 69	<13	13 - 17	18 - 23	24 - 34	35+

Activity 3   **1 Mile Walk Test**

Activity Description

A variety of walking and running test protocols exist that can be used to estimate the cardiorespiratory fitness of an individual. These field tests require minimal equipment and can accommodate individuals of varying ages and fitness levels. Walking is a basic human movement the vast majority of the population can execute safely. Running, on the other hand, is more challenging and for many adults not something executed frequently, if at all. Run/walk field tests require the user to walk or run as fast as possible over a set distance or for a predetermined period of time. Individuals with adequate fitness should perform timed tests, whereas deconditioned individuals may require pacing over a set distance.

Like other sub-max protocols, field tests for cardiorespiratory fitness rely on the correlation between sub-max workload and heart rates. The assessment capitalizes on the increased oxygen demand of the body to determine fitness level. The estimation of VO_2 relies on the average speed to complete the assessment and the heart rate response to the activity.

The 1 Mile Walk Test requires the subject to walk as fast as possible on a measured track or flat mile course. Heart rate is measured at the end of the test and this value is used to predict VO_2max (ml/kg/min). An additional benefit to this assessment is that it can be administered to a single subject or a group of subjects at the same time.

Procedures

The following activity involves administering the 1 Mile Walk Test on a volunteer subject. Be sure to read through the entire lab prior to implementing this assessment.

Step 1   *Preparation.* Ensure that the subject:
1. Has signed a consent form and has been cleared to participate in activity
2. Has been checked for fitness preparation (Activity 1)
3. Is wearing appropriate clothes for activity
4. Has performed a general warm-up

Step 2   *Stop Test Indicators.* Read and explain the following Stop Test Indicators to the subject.

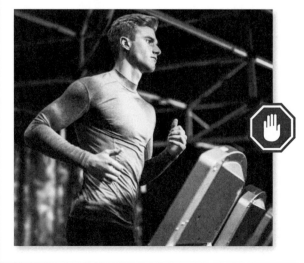

Indications for Test Termination

- Subject no longer feels comfortable doing the test.
- Subject's skin becomes pale.
- Subject fails to keep cadence for 20 seconds or more.
- Subject has an inability to focus attention.
- Subject experiences faintness, dizziness, or lightheadedness.
- Subject experiences upset stomach or vomiting symptoms.
- Subject experiences dysfunction in breathing.
- Subject experiences chest pain.
- Subject experiences side stitch, cramp, strain, fatigue.

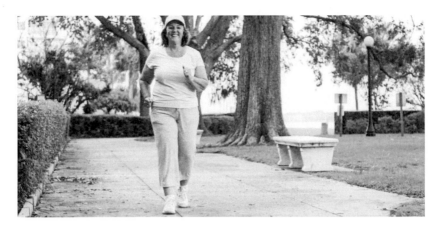

Step 3 **Warm-Up.** Have the subject warm-up by walking at a comfortable pace.

Step 4 **Stretch.** Have the subject stretch thoroughly.

Step 5 **Review Procedures.** Explain the test protocol and answer any questions.

Step 6 **Test Start.** Have the subject ready him or herself behind the beginning mark of the measured mile. Timer begins with a "Ready, Go," signal and starts the watch as the subject begins walking, as fast as possible, through the measured course. You may want to provide the time at each lap, as well as encouragement of effort to enhance test validity.

Step 7 **Test Finish.** At the end of the measured mile (4 laps on standard track) you call out the time to the subject as they cross the measured mile marker and record the number below.

   One mile walk time _____

Step 8 **Palpate Heart Rate.** At the conclusion of the walk test immediately assess the subject's pulse for **15 seconds**. A ten second heart rate can be used to more accurately assess the actual heart rate during the activity, as the heart rate will decline as soon as the activity is stopped.

   15 second heart rate _____ *beats*

Step 9 **Calculate 60 second Heart Rate.** Record the subject's 15 second heart rate and then calculate the subject's 60 second heart rate by multiplying the 15 second value by 4 (or 10-second value by 6).

   15 second heart rate _____ *x 4 =* _____ *beats/min*

Step 10 **Cool down.** Have the subject perform a cool down at the completion of the activity.

Procedures for Estimating VO$_2$max

Step 1 **Organize Data.** To calculate the subject's fitness level (VO$_2$) you will need to have the subject or client's age, current body weight, and sex (this information should have already been gathered during the initial screening process). The information gathered from the performance of the test should be transferred to the following data-recording sheet.

Age	Weight	Sex	One Mile Walk Time	Calculated 60-second heart rate (Step 9)

Step 2 *Calculate fitness level score.* The following formula is used to calculate VO$_2$max (ml/kg/min) for the 1 Mile Walk Test from the recorded information. Using the equation template that follows, calculate the estimated VO$_2$.

Calculating VO$_2$max

VO$_2$max (ml/kg/min) = 132.853 − 0.0769(weight) − 0.3877(age) + 6.315(gender) − 3.2649(time) − 0.1565(Heart Rate)

- **Weight** is in pounds
- **Age** is in years
- **Sex** = 0 for females and 1 for males
- **Time** is in minutes and hundredths of minutes *(ex. 13.31 = 13 minutes and 31 seconds)*
  - divide 31 seconds by 60 seconds
- **Heart rate** is in beats per minute

0.0769 x _____ lbs. = _____ Value #1

0.3877 x _____ years = _____ Value #2

6.3150 x _____ sex = _____ Value #3

3.2649 x _____ min. = _____ Value #4

0.1565 x _____ HR = _____ Value #5

132.853 − (Value #1) − (Value #2) + (Value #3) − (Value #4) − (Value #5) = _____ ml/kg/min

In the space provided, calculate the subject's estimated VO$_2$max (ml/kg/min) from the 1 Mile Walk Test results.

132.853 − (_____ #1) − (_____ #2) + (_____ #3) − (_____ #4) − (_____ #5) = _____ ml/kg/min

Predicted VO$_2$max _____ *ml/kg/min*

Evaluating Results

To determine the cardiovascular fitness, match the predicted VO$_2$max results by sex, as follows:

Aerobic Fitness Classification for the General Population (ml · kg^{-1} · min^{-1})						Aerobic Fitness Classification for the General Population (ml · kg^{-1} · min^{-1})					
MEN						WOMEN					
Age (Years)	20-29	30-39	40-49	50-59	60+	Age (Years)	20-29	30-39	40-49	50-59	60+
Above Average	>46.8	>44.6	>41.8	>38.5	>35.3	Above Average	>38.1	>36.7	>33.8	>30.9	>29.4
Average	42.5 – 46.7	41.0 – 44.5	38.1 – 41.7	35.2 – 38.4	31.8 – 35.2	Average	35.2 – 38	33.9 – 36.6	30.9 – 33.7	28.3 – 30.8	25.9 – 29.3
Below Average	<42.4	<40.9	<38	<35.1	<31.7	Below Average	<35.1	<33.8	<30.8	<28.2	<25.8

Cardiorespiratory Fitness Testing

Activity 4 **1.5 Mile Run Test**

Activity Description

Similar to the 1 Mile Walk Test, administration protocols for the 1.5 Mile Run Test requires the subject to travel a set distance for time to predict VO_2max. The difference in protocol is the assessment results are based on time-to-completion rather than time and heart rate response so the subject must jog/run the 1.5 miles as fast as possible on a measured track for accurate results. The total time used to complete the distance is converted into an estimated VO_2max using calculations. Like the walk test, this assessment can be administered with a single subject or a group at the same time. A major difference between walking and running tests is the role effort plays in the test outcome. Individuals that do not put forth a maximal effort will receive a score that underpredicts their actual oxygen efficiency. Additionally, running tests are used for healthy individuals with previous running experience and practice with the distance covered. New exercisers should avoid maximal run tests as their risk for a negative outcome is elevated and the data will likely be skewed due to poor economy and inaccurate pacing.

Procedures

The following activity requires the administration of the 1.5 Mile Run Test with a test subject. Be sure to read through the entire lab prior to implementing this assessment.

Step 1 *Preparation.* Ensure that the subject:
1. Has signed a consent form and has been cleared to participate in activity
2. Has been checked for fitness preparation (Activity 1)
3. Is wearing appropriate clothes for activity
4. Has performed a general warm-up

Step 2 *Stop Test Indicators.* Read and explain the following Stop Test Indicators to the subject.

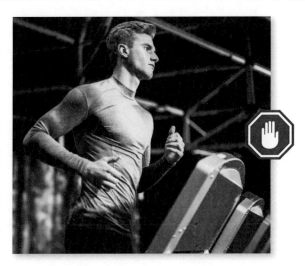

Indications for Test Termination

- Subject no longer feels comfortable doing the test.
- Subject's skin becomes pale.
- Subject fails to keep cadence for 20 seconds or more.
- Subject has an inability to focus attention.
- Subject experiences faintness, dizziness, or lightheadedness.
- Subject experiences upset stomach or vomiting symptoms.
- Subject experiences dysfunction in breathing.
- Subject experiences chest pain.
- Subject experiences side stitch, cramp, strain, fatigue.

Step 3 *Warm-Up.* Have the subject warm-up with some slow jogging for 3-5 minutes.

Step 4 *Stretch.* Have the subject stretch thoroughly.

Step 5 **Review Procedures.** Explain the purpose of the test to the subject and answer any questions they may have regarding the procedure. Clearly inform the test subject that they are to run/jog 6 laps (1.5 miles on a standard track) or the full distance of the course as fast as possible.

Step 6 **Test Prep.** Have the test subject stand behind the starting line of the measured distance.

Step 7 **Test Start.** Timer begins with a "Ready, Go" signal and starts the stopwatch as the test subject begins running the 1.5 mile distance.

Step 8 **Monitor.** When the test subject passes the start/stop line, inform him or her of the lap number they are on and the time. Look for signs of physical distress throughout the duration of the test.

Step 9 **Test Finish.** At the completion of lap 6, or 1.5 miles, the timer calls out the participant's time and records it.

  Record 1.5 mile run time here _____

Procedures for Estimating VO$_2$max

Step 1 **Review of Formula.** Calculating the fitness level (estimated VO$_2$max) from the subject's 1.5 mile run time involves the use of the following formula:

$$VO_2 = \text{horizontal velocity m/min} \times \frac{0.2 \text{ ml/kg/min}}{\text{m/min}} + 3.5 \text{ ml/kg/min}$$

Step 2 **Finding horizontal run speed in (m/min).** The formula is not as complicated as it appears. The first thing that must be determined is the average horizontal running velocity of the subject in meters per minute. To do this you must convert the distance completed into meters and divide it by the number of minutes it took to complete the full distance.

Example

> **Meter Conversion**
> 1.5 miles = 2,413.8 meters
> 2,413.8 must then be divided by the time it took to complete the run, in minutes *(use whole numbers)*
>
> **Seconds conversion**
> If it took 12:13 to complete the run, the divisor would be 12.21
> Or {12 min + (13/60 seconds)} = 12 min + (0.21 seconds)
>
> **(m/min) conversion**
> If it took 12:00 minutes to complete the run the horizontal velocity would be 201.15
> 2,413.8 m / 12 min. = 201.15 m/min (horizontal velocity)
>
> Perform your conversion below:
>
>   *2,413.8 meters ÷* _____ *minutes =* _____ *m/min (horizontal velocity)*

Step 3 **VO$_2$max Conversion.** Calculate the subject's estimated VO$_2$max. Consider the previous example:

Example VO$_2$max conversion

$$VO_2 = \text{horizontal velocity m/min} \times \frac{0.2 \text{ ml/kg/min}}{\text{m/min}} + 3.5 \text{ ml/kg/min}$$

$$VO_2 = 201 \text{ m/min} \times \frac{0.2 \text{ ml/kg/min}}{\text{m/min}} + 3.5 \text{ ml/kg/min}$$

$$VO_2 = 43.7 \text{ ml/kg/min}$$

Perform your conversion below:

$$VO_2 = \underline{\hspace{2cm}} \text{ horizontal velocity m/min} \times \frac{0.2 \text{ ml/kg/min}}{\text{m/min}} + 3.5 \text{ ml/kg/min}$$

$$VO_2 = \underline{\hspace{2cm}} \text{ ml/kg/min}$$

The following chart can also be used as a quick reference:

1.5 Mile Time	VO$_2$max ml/kg/min	1.5 Mile Time	VO$_2$max ml/kg/min	1.5 Mile Time	VO$_2$max ml/kg/min
<7:31	75	14:01 – 14:30	34	15:01 – 15:30	31
7:31 – 8:00	72	14:31 – 15:00	33	15:31 – 16:00	30
8:01 – 8:30	67	11:01 – 11:30	46	16:01 – 16:30	28
8:31 – 9:00	62	11:31 – 12:00	44	16:31 – 17:00	27
9:01 – 9:30	58	12:01 – 12:30	41	17:01 – 17:30	26
9:31 – 10:00	55	12:31 – 13:00	39	17:31 – 18:00	25
10:01 – 10:30	52	13:01 – 13:30	37		
10:31 – 11:00	49	13:31 – 14:00	36		

To determine the cardiovascular fitness, match the predicted VO$_2$max results by sex, as follows:

Aerobic Fitness Classification for the General Population (ml · kg^{-1} · min^{-1})						Aerobic Fitness Classification for the General Population (ml · kg^{-1} · min^{-1})					
MEN						WOMEN					
Age (Years)	20-29	30-39	40-49	50-59	60+	Age (Years)	20-29	30-39	40-49	50-59	60+
Above Average	>46.8	>44.6	>41.8	>38.5	>35.3	Above Average	>38.1	>36.7	>33.8	>30.9	>29.4
Average	42.5 – 46.7	41.0 – 44.5	38.1 – 41.7	35.2 – 38.4	31.8 – 35.2	Average	35.2 – 38	33.9 – 36.6	30.9 – 33.7	28.3 – 30.8	25.9 – 29.3
Below Average	<42.4	<40.9	<38	<35.1	<31.7	Below Average	<35.1	<33.8	<30.8	<28.2	<25.8

Cardiorespiratory Fitness Testing Quiz

1. Which of the following tests would be inappropriate for a deconditioned or older client?

    _____ a. The 1 mile walk test
    _____ b. The 3 minute step test
    _____ c. The 1.5 mile run test
    _____ d. All of the above should not be used with older clients

2. True or False? Recovery heart rate assessed following the 1 mile walk test can be used in a formula to predict VO_2max.

    _____ a. True
    _____ b. False

3. Which of the following tests for CRF requires a metronome for specific pacing during the effort?

    _____ a. 1.5 mile run test
    _____ b. 3 minute step test
    _____ c. 1 mile walk test
    _____ d. 12 minute swim test

4. Which of the following is not a stop test indicator?

    _____ a. The subject's skin becomes pale
    _____ b. The subject experiences light chest pain
    _____ c. The subject fails to keep cadence for 8 seconds or more
    _____ d. The subject has an inability to focus

5. The client's RPE during the 3 minute step test should not exceed _____ on the 1-10 RPE scale.

    _____ a. 4
    _____ b. 6
    _____ c. 7
    _____ d. 9

6. All of the following are needed to calculate VO_2max from the Rockport One Mile Walk Test, except?

    ____ a. Body weight in pounds
    ____ b. Minutes of activity performed
    ____ c. Participant's sex
    ____ d. mL of oxygen used

7. Which of the following is used to estimate a VO_2max value when implementing the 1.5 mile test?

    ____ a. Heart rate
    ____ b. Blood pressure
    ____ c. RPE
    ____ d. Time to completion

8. A 35 year-old female with a VO_2max of 35 ml/kg/min would have an aerobic fitness classification of:

    ____ a. Below average
    ____ b. Average
    ____ c. Above average
    ____ d. Diseased

9. Which of the following statements related to the 1.5 mile run test is not correct?

    ____ a. Time-to-completion is used to estimate VO_2max
    ____ b. RPE measures should range from 5-8 on a 1-10 RPE scale
    ____ c. New exercises should not use this test due to poor economy
    ____ d. Inaccurate pacing will greatly impact test validity

10. Which of the following is addressed by a fitness test preparation checklist?

    ____ a. Making sure all equipment is calibrated and working correctly
    ____ b. Checking to make sure the subject can recognize stop test indicators
    ____ c. Making sure the subject has performed an appropriate warm-up
    ____ d. All of the above

◆ Muscular Fitness Testing

This lab corresponds to the following text – Chapter 7: pages 319-321, 326-328, 330

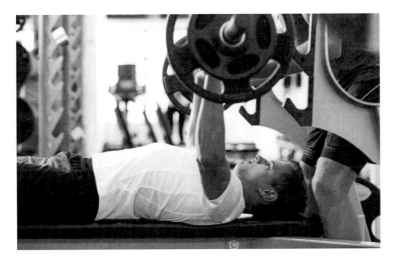

Activity 1 **Multi-Repetition Bench Press**

Activity Description

Although muscular strength is defined as the force that a muscle or muscle group can voluntarily exert against a resistance in one maximal effort, it is often neither safe nor practical to have individuals perform one repetition maximum (1RM) assessments. Similar to cardiorespiratory fitness tests, maximum capabilities can be estimated through a formula based on measurements using a submaximal load. Strength assessments using multiple repetition tests are commonly performed on cross-joint movements such as the squat, deadlift, leg press, row, and bench press. The cross-joint assessment increases the use of stabilization from contributing musculature which is often the determining factor in maximal force output when performing free weight movements.

Multi-repetition testing can be a safe and effective way to evaluate and monitor strength gains. Although it does not require a person to perform a 1RM, there is a close relationship between the amount of weight a person can lift one time and the amount of weight that they can lift a few times. To maintain a high correlation between 1RM and multi-repetition predictions, the strength tests should be limited to no more than 10 repetitions and no fewer than 3 repetitions. Staying within this range will help ensure safety and test validity. The following activity requires the performance of a repetition test using the free weight bench press to determine a 1RM for a test subject. The assessment protocols can be applied to any number of free weight movements and are valuable to predict training intensities as well as track and monitor program effectiveness. The bench press is chosen for this activity because it is a good indicator of overall upper body strength as it involves the synergistic actions of shoulder horizontal adduction and arm extension. Additionally, because it is a free weight movement, it calls upon the stabilizing properties of the associated musculature.

The accuracy of strength testing is subject to several factors. The primary factor is the role of the nervous system. Since the performance of maximal muscle contractions is nervous-system dependent, it is important to consider emotional and mental factors before performing tests to assess muscular strength. Other factors which may be considered include daily fatigue, energy system capacity, and hydration status. In tests requiring short duration and maximal contractions, blood supply is not a limiting factor because the role of oxygen is de-emphasized during energy metabolism for short-burst activities. It is important to note that if a person is new to exercise, strength testing, albeit free weight or machine, may be unwarranted until a baseline level of strength, stability, and movement proficiency is developed. This can take a few sessions to acquire. One should also avoid exposing a person to high physical demands if they have never performed resistance training before, as excessive soreness and injury can result.

Equipment

- Free weight bench press
- Free weight
- 45 lb. Olympic bar (lighter bars can be substituted)
- Safety clips

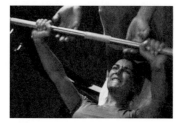

Procedures

Strength is measured using units of force or torque. These units may be expressed as pounds (lb.), kilograms (kg), or newtons (N). For this lab we will be using pounds as the unit of force. Prior to testing, determine a weight that can be lifted for approximately five repetitions. If an individual cannot perform at least 15 modified push-ups (female) or 20 conventional push-ups (male), they should not perform this test. In addition, the test should not be used if it is the first time the subject has performed the bench press technique.

Step 1 **Warm-up.** Make sure that the subject has performed an adequate warm-up and is prepared for the test using the test preparation checklist. The technician should always inspect the equipment prior to each test to be sure it is in proper working condition.

Step 2 **Protocol Review.** (Review Steps #3 - #6) Have the test subject perform two or three progressive intensity trials to ensure his or her form is perfect and that the subject is comfortable with the equipment. This will also act as a specific warm-up, increasing neural preparation and movement efficiency.

Step 3 **Ready Position.** Have the individual lie in the supine position on a flat bench with feet flat on the floor. Be sure the body lines up appropriately with the bench. The subject should not be too far forward or too far back on the bench (normal alignment is eyes under the bar). The technician should be directly behind the bar, attentive, and in a position to safely manage the bar movement.

Step 4 **Lift Off.** Instruct the subject to signal you when he or she is ready to lift the bar. Have them lift the bar off the rack under assistance. Their arms should be fully extended with the bar positioned over the chest. Instruct the subject to maintain the starting position as you release support on the bar.

Step 5 **Downward Movement Phase.** In the eccentric movement phase, the subject lowers the bar to his or her chest in a controlled manner. Instruct the subject to maintain strict body position and to keep the wrists straight. Once the bar contacts the chest, or the terminal range of motion (ROM) is reached, the bar should be transitioned upward without bouncing off the subject's chest.

Step 6 **Upward Movement Phase.** During the concentric movement phase, the subject will push the bar upward to full elbow extension. Instruct them to maintain body position without arching the back or lifting the glutes off the bench. Be sure the subject pushes the bar up evenly.

Step 7 **Movement Repetition.** Repeat steps 5 and 6 (downward and upward movement phases) until muscular failure is reached and the subject cannot complete another repetition. Safely re-rack the bar and then record results on the Data Recording Sheet.

Weight _____   *Repetitions* _____

*** **Danger** ***

It is important to closely monitor each repetition for volitional fatigue or improper body mechanics. If the individual shows signs of stability fatigue or an inability to maintain posture – stop the test and rerack the weight. Also, be sure the subject is breathing correctly during each repetition, inhaling during the eccentric and exhaling during the concentric movement.

Step 8 *Calculate 1RM from Results.* Using the formula below, calculate the estimated 1RM using the weight lifted and the number of repetitions completed. Record the results on the data recording form.

Example
A male performs 5 repetitions to failure using 150 lb.

3% Formula
$[(0.03 \times \text{repetitions attained}) + 1.0] \times \text{weight used}$
Estimated 1RM = $[(0.03 \times 5 \text{ repetitions}) + 1.0] \times 150$ lb.
Estimated 1RM = $1.15 \times 150 = 172.5$ lb.

MULTI-REPETITION STRENGTH DATA RECORDING FORM

Name: _____   Date: _____

   Sex: _____   Age: _____   Body Weight: _____ lb. _____ kg

   Exercise Assessed: _____

      Resistance used: _____ lb.   Repetitions Performed: _____

Multi-Repetition Formula

$[(0.03 \times \text{repetitions performed } _____) + 1.0] \times \text{weight used } _____$ lb.

[_____ + 1.0] x _____ lb.

Bench Press Score = _____ lb.

Step 9 *Interpret Results.* The table that follows illustrates Relative Bench Press Strength Norms based on body weight in both males and females. To find your subject's strength classification divide the subject's calculated 1RM by his or her current body weight.

Weight lifted ÷ body weight = upper body strength rating

_____ weight lifted ÷ _____ body weight = _____ upper body strength rating

Upper Body Strength Rating _____

Relative Bench Press Strength Norms

Age (Years)	20-29		30-39		40-49		50-59		60 +	
Classification	M	F	M	F	M	F	M	F	M	F
Above Average	>1.17	>.72	>1.01	>.62	>.91	>.57	>.81	>.51	>.74	>.51
Average	.97 - 1.16	.59 - .71	.86 - 1.00	.53 - .61	.78 - .90	.48 - .56	.70 - .80	.43 - .50	.63 - .73	.41 - .50
Below Average	<.96	<.58	<.85	<.52	<.77	<.47	<.69	<.42	<.62	<.40

Activity 2 **Push-up Test / Modified Push-up Test**

Activity Description

Muscular strength and endurance are interrelated but differ in the amount of force produced to accomplish a task. Muscular endurance is defined as the ability of the muscle to contract repeatedly while resisting fatigue over a prolonged period of time. Often referred to as localized muscular endurance, the ability of a muscle to continue to produce force to maintain an activity is dependent upon the strength of the muscle itself, as well as the stabilizers that support the movement. Muscles that are weak do not maintain the ability to perform repetitive contractions when the force demands increase. This limits the ability of the body to perform beneficial activities and may become an obstacle to improving physical fitness.

A very popular method to assess upper body endurance is the push-up test. It has classically been one of the primary field tests used to measure upper body endurance among individuals and groups. The test provides an accurate assessment of endurance if performed correctly. Therefore, it is extremely important for the test subject to adhere to proper movement technique, as test validity is negatively affected if correct form is not maintained. Many individuals do not possess the trunk strength to maintain the proper posture while performing the pressing movement from the ground. For this reason, the push-up test is often subject to tester discretion which can again cause test validity to be skewed. To accurately assess anaerobic endurance capacity, each repetition must be performed with exacting technique throughout the duration of the test.

> **Note:** Although the push-up test is designed as an anaerobic endurance assessment, it can become a measure of anaerobic muscular strength when people do not possess the ability to perform multiple repetitions with proper form. When the test subject's muscles are only able to generate enough force to complete a few repetitions the test is actually identifying anaerobic strength rather than anaerobic endurance.

Procedures

The push-up test requires a subject to perform a maximal number of repetitions in the allotted time period. For this test, 60 seconds will be used. The subject may reach failure early in the test. If this occurs, they may rest in the starting position until they are able to perform additional repetitions. If an individual fails to perform the repetitions with the appropriate form through a complete ROM, the test should be stopped. Other reasons for disqualification include failure to maintain body position or an inability to move the entire body through the required ROM. Incorrect movements should not be scored. If the subject fails to perform the movement correctly for more than three repetitions, they should be asked to stop the test.

Prior to testing, the test subject should be instructed on proper movement technique and practice the test. As in any exercise test, they should meet the pre-test requirements of the test checklist. Following an adequate warm-up, the subject should perform the technique for a minimum of 3-4 repetitions to ensure their ability and technique allow for safe testing procedures. If they cannot perform or are unable to follow the instructions listed below, they should not be tested using the assessment protocol. The execution technique varies slightly for males and females. Be sure to read through each description and implement the proper sex-specific assessment protocols.

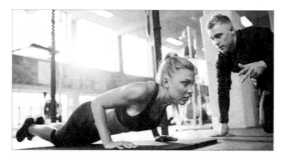

Push-up (Males)

Step 1 **Test Setup.** Select an area with a solid, flat surface. Make sure that the area selected is in an environment that is safe and free of hazards. You may want to place a gym mat on the ground in an area that offers enough space for the assessment to be performed safely.

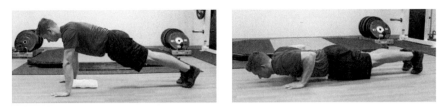

Step 2 **Starting Position.** Have the subject lie prone on the floor with his body extended. Place the hands approximately shoulder-width apart with thumbs located under the shoulders. The feet should be no more than 6" apart. Have the subject lift the body to a point where the arms are extended, and the body is in proper alignment (do not allow the subject to perform hip extension or hip flexion during any phase of the movement). Place a towel rolled to approximately 3 inches beneath the chest at 90° of flexion.

Step 3 **Begin Assessment.** Once the subject is in position, the technician should give the "Go" command and begin timing. The subject should lower themselves in a rigid straight position down to the towel, the point at which their elbows are at approximately 90° of flexion.

Step 4 **Movement Repetition.** The subject returns to the extended arm position by pushing upward until the elbows are fully extended. This movement should be performed until volitional failure, technique breakdown occurs, or the full 60 second duration of the test is completed. Count out loud each repetition the subject completes correctly.

> **Note:** During the execution of the test be sure that the subject performs the movement through a full ROM at the shoulder and elbow. It is common to limit ROM during arm flexion and extension to try and achieve a higher score. It is also important that the subject maintains a rigid body position. At no time should the spine/torso be placed in a flexed or hyperextended position.

Common mechanical performance errors include:

- Excessive scapular protraction and retraction without adequate elbow flexion
- Scapular elevation
- Excessive humeral abduction
- Hip flexion or hip and back extension
- Incorrect wrist to elbow relationship
- Incorrect hand placement including inward rotation

Step 5 **Data Collection/Recording.** Record the number of repetitions successfully performed in one minute on the Data Recording Sheet.

Step 6 **Interpret Results.** The chart at the end of the lab illustrates Push-up Testing Norms for both males and females within each age category.

Modified Push-up (Females)

Step 1 ***Starting Position.*** The technique is modified for female subjects so that their knees are the first point of contact with the ground as opposed to the feet in the standard push-up position. This technique shortens the resistance arm which reduces the load placed upon the movement. The female subject begins by lying prone on the floor with the body extended. Have the subject place their hands approximately shoulder-width apart with the thumbs placed directly under the shoulders. The feet and knees should be together or no more than 6" apart. To help maintain rigid body position during the execution of the test, the subject can flex the knees to 90°. This technique helps to reduce spinal hyperextension (sagging hips), which is often performed during push-ups from the knees. Have the subject lift the body to a point where the arms are completely extended. The legs should be in the bent-knee position with the body straight from the shoulders to the knees. A mat may be used to reduce the discomfort of knee contact with the ground. Place a towel rolled to approximately 3 inches beneath the chest at 90° of flexion.

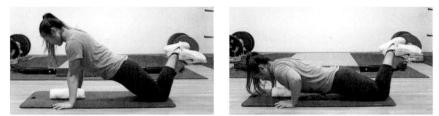

Step 2 ***Begin Assessment.*** Once the correct position is established the technician should give the "Go" command and begin timing. The subject should lower themselves in a rigid, straight position down to a point at which the elbows are at approximately 90° of flexion and the body reaches the towel.

Step 3 ***Movement Repetition.*** The subject returns to the extended arm position by pushing upward until the elbows are fully extended. The subject may rest in the arm extended position, if necessary, during the assessment. This movement should be performed until volitional failure, technique breakdown, or the full duration of the test is completed. Count out loud each repetition the subject completes correctly.

> **Note:** During the execution of the test be sure that the subject performs the movement through a full ROM. It is common for a test subject to limit arm flexion and extension ROM to try and achieve a higher score. It is also important that the subject maintains rigid body position. At no time should the spine/torso be placed in a flexed or hyperextended position.

Common mechanical performance errors include:

- Excessive scapular protraction and retraction without adequate elbow flexion
- Scapular elevation
- Excessive humeral abduction
- Hip flexion or hip and back extension
- Incorrect wrist to elbow relationship
- Incorrect hand placement including inward rotation

Step 4 ***Data Collection/Recording.*** Record the number of repetitions successfully performed in one minute on the Data Recording Sheet.

Step 5 ***Interpret Results.*** The following chart illustrates Push-up Testing Norms for both males and females within each age category.

PUSH-UP TEST RECORDING FORM

Name: _____   Date: _____

Sex: _____   Age: _____

Repetitions completed: _____   Fitness Rating: _____

	Classifications for Push-up Test						
	Age (Years)	15-19	20-29	30-39	40-49	50-59	60-69
Men	Above Average	>28	>28	>21	>16	>12	>10
	Average	22-28	21-28	17-21	13-16	10-12	8-10
	Below Average	<22	<21	<17	<13	<10	<8
Women	Above Average	>24	>20	>19	>14	>11	>10
	Average	18-24	15-20	13-19	11-14	7-11	5-10
	Below Average	<18	<15	<13	<11	<7	<5

Activity 3 **Abdominal Curl-up Test**

Activity Description

The muscles of the core and abdomen are predominately comprised of slow-twitch muscle fibers. They are highly resistant to fatigue due to their constant responsibility in postural stabilization. The maintenance of adequate trunk strength and endurance are extremely important factors for healthy posture, the performance of general physical activity, and lower back health.

Historically, the sit-up was the most widely-used muscle endurance test in fitness assessments. Modern literature has identified that the full sit-up employs hip flexion for 60° of the traditional movement and are increasingly involved when an individual's feet are held down by an outside force. The recommended alternative to the full sit-up is an abdominal curl-up or crunch, which is defined as trunk flexion up to approximately 30°. This type of half sit-up isolates the abdominal musculature better than any other type of sit-up studied. These facts have led to the use of the abdominal curl-up for better assessment of abdominal endurance. Numerous versions of the abdominal curl-up test have been developed over the last two decades as curl-up tests have become the dominant field test of muscular endurance. Some of these tests include the Canadian partial curl-up, the Fit Youth Today (FYT) curl-up, the Modified trunk-curl, the Georgia Tech (GTCU) curl-up, and the Bench trunk-curl (BTC). The test for this lab is based upon endurance capabilities using a set pace. The test requires the subject to repetitively contract the abdominal musculature at a metronome paced 20 curl-ups per minute (40 beats/min) for as many repetitions as possible, up to a maximum of 75. Each repetition should be performed in a controlled fashion to the pace set by the metronome. As soon as the subject cannot continue at the metronome pace, the test is stopped.

Equipment

- Stopwatch   • Gym mat   • Metronome

Procedures

The test requires a subject to perform a maximal number of repetitions at a set pace. Some individuals may reach failure early in the test. If this occurs, the test is stopped, and the score is recorded. If an individual fails to perform the repetitions with a full ROM or cannot maintain the 3 second per contraction pace they should stop the test. Incorrect movements should not be scored, this includes creating momentum from the floor to attain a mechanical advantage. If the subject fails to perform the movement correctly for more than three repetitions, they should be asked to stop the test.

Prior to testing, the subject should be instructed on proper movement technique. As in any test, he or she should meet the pre-test requirements of the test checklist. Following an adequate warm-up, the subject should perform the technique for a minimum of 3-4 repetitions to ensure that their ability and movement technique allow for safe testing protocols. If they cannot perform or are unable to follow the instructions listed below, he or she should not be tested.

Step 1   *Test Set Up.* Select an area with a solid flat surface. Make sure that the area selected is safe and the surrounding environment is appropriate for testing. Place a gym mat on the ground in an area that offers enough space for the assessment.

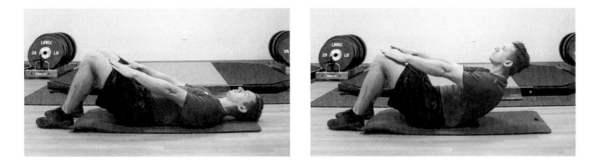

Step 2   *Starting Position.* Have the test subject assume the supine position with knees flexed and feet flat on the floor approximately 12" apart. The arms should be extended, palms resting on the thighs with fingertips pointing at the knees.

Step 3   *Begin Assessment.* Set the metronome for 40 beats/min. On the "Go" command, the subject curls-up in a controlled manner until the fingers reach the top of the knees as the cadence sounds. Each beat represents a transitional change in the movement. The movements should be controlled and on pace with the metronome.

Step 4   *Movement Repetition.* The subject then returns to the starting position until the upper back contacts the mat while the abdominals remain contracted. This should be repeated until the subject cannot perform any more repetitions through the full ROM, or the time expires.

Step 5   *Data Collection.* The technician should count out loud each correctly-performed repetition. If the subject performs 75 repetitions, stop the test and record the results. Subjects stopping before the terminal score of 75 repetitions should have their score recorded at the end of the test.

Step 6   *Interpretation of Results.* The following table indicates the endurance ratings for trunk flexion for both males and females. It is based on the number of completed curl-ups for each age category. The table should be used to help interpret the test score.

CURL-UP TEST RECORDING FORM

Name: _____   Date: _____

Sex: _____   Age: _____

Repetitions completed: _____   Fitness Rating: _____

Classification for Abdominal Curl-up Test						
	Age (Years)	20-29	30-39	40-49	50-59	60-69
Men	Above Average	>21	>18	>18	>17	>16
	Average	16 - 20	15 - 17	13 - 17	11 - 16	11 - 15
	Below Average	<16	<15	<13	<11	<11
Women	Above Average	>18	>19	>19	>19	>17
	Average	14 - 17	11 - 18	11 - 18	10 - 18	8 - 16
	Below Average	<14	<11	<11	<10	<8

Muscular Fitness Testing Lab Quiz

1. True or False? It is recommended to perform 1RM assessments with clients seeking to improve their muscular strength as these tests provide the highest accuracy.

    ____ a. True
    ____ b. False

2. To maintain a high correlation between 1RM and multi-repetition predictions, strength tests should be limited to no more than ____ repetitions.

    ____ a. 5
    ____ b. 7
    ____ c. 10
    ____ d. 15

3. Which system is the primary determinant of outcomes during a strength assessment?

    ____ a. Cardiovascular
    ____ b. Nervous
    ____ c. Metabolic
    ____ d. Endocrine

4. Which of the following potentially indicates a client should not perform the multi-rep bench press test?

    ____ a. The client is male and can only complete 10 conventional push-ups
    ____ b. The client is female and has limited experience bench pressing
    ____ c. The client has not bench pressed for more than three months
    ____ d. All the above

5. If a client performs 8 repetitions using 200 lb. during the multi-rep bench press test, what would be their estimated 1RM?

    ____ a. 225 lb.
    ____ b. 235 lb.
    ____ c. 248 lb.
    ____ d. 264 lb.

6. _____ is defined as the ability of the muscle to contract repeatedly while resisting fatigue over a prolonged period of time.

    _____ a. Muscular strength
    _____ b. Muscular power
    _____ c. Muscular endurance
    _____ d. Muscular hypertrophy

7. What is the duration of the push-up test?

    _____ a. 45 seconds
    _____ b. 60 seconds
    _____ c. 75 seconds
    _____ d. 120 seconds

8. Which of the following is not a common error during the push-up or modified push-up test?

    _____ a. Incorrect hand placement
    _____ b. Excessive scapular protraction
    _____ c. Excessive elbow extension
    _____ d. Hip flexion and extension

9. What is the terminal number of repetitions used for the abdominal curl-up test?

    _____ a. 50
    _____ b. 65
    _____ c. 75
    _____ d. 95

10. Why has the abdominal curl-up movement replaced the traditional sit-up movement for assessment of muscular endurance in the trunk?

    _____ a. The sit-up requires excess activation of the hip flexors
    _____ b. The sit-up is too difficult for most people to perform
    _____ c. The sit-up movement requires excess activation of the erector spinae
    _____ d. All of the above are correct

◆ Flexibility and Mobility Testing

This lab corresponds to the following text – Chapter 7: Pages 336-345

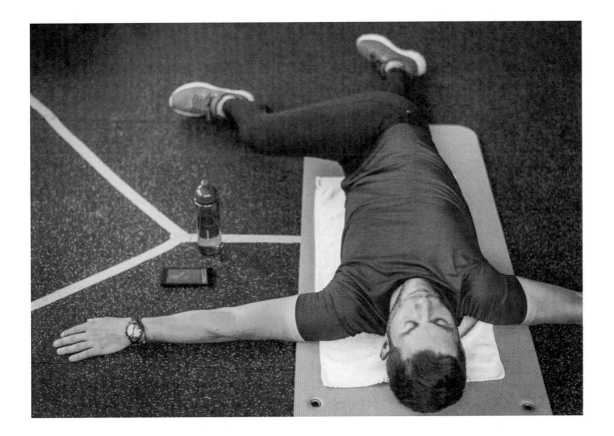

Activity 1 **Assessing Flexibility**

Activity Description

This lab employs field flexibility assessments for primary joint structures. Performance of these assessments can provide the exercise professional with valuable information pertaining to the subject's range of motion (ROM) capabilities and subsequent needs. The assessments serve to establish a baseline of flexibility and provide information about the client's movement capabilities and limitations. Arguably, the most valuable information pertaining to movement restrictions will occur during the actual observation of the subject's performance of each activity.

Procedures

Read through the six field flexibility assessments in your textbook (pages 338-343). Have your volunteer subject perform an adequate warm-up prior to starting the assessment battery. Once the test subject is appropriately prepared, have them perform each assessment technique. Be sure to perform a bilateral assessment where applicable, as ROM differences between contralateral joints are common. Report your findings at the end of this section on the recording form. Remember to be as detailed as possible when reporting your findings.

Note: Instruct the subject to perform the movements in a controlled fashion and not to attempt to forcibly attain a position outside of his or her functional ROM.

FLEXIBILITY ASSESSMENT RECORDING FORM

Name: _____ Date: _____

1. **Apley Back Scratch Test** *(page 338)*

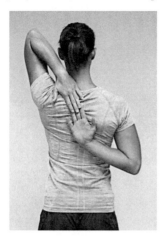

Observation	Score
Fingers are touching	1 - Good
Fingers are not touching but less than two inches apart	2 – Borderline
Fingertips are greater than two inches apart	3 – Needs work

Assessed Structures: _____

_____

Left Score _____ Right Score _____

Notes: _____

2. **Modified Thomas Test** *(page 339)*

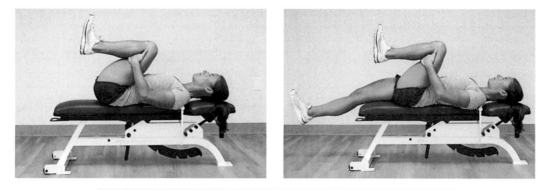

Observation	Score
Straight leg or flexed knee contact with bench	1 - Good
Hamstring <1 inch	2 – Borderline
Hamstring >1 inch	3 – Needs work

Assessed Structures: _____

_____

Left Score _____ Right Score _____

Notes: _____

3. **Trunk Extension Test** *(page 340)*

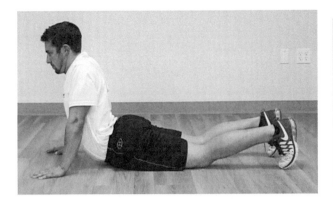

Scoring with suprasternal notch measurement	
Excellent	> 12 inches (30 cm)
Good	> 8 inches (20 cm)
Fair	> 4 inches (10 cm)
Scoring with Iliac crest measurement	
Good	Hips remain on the ground
Borderline	< 1 inch (2.54 cm)
Needs work	> 1 inch (2.54 cm)

Assessed Structures: _____

_____

Score _____

Notes: _____

4. **Trunk Flexion Test** *(page 341)*

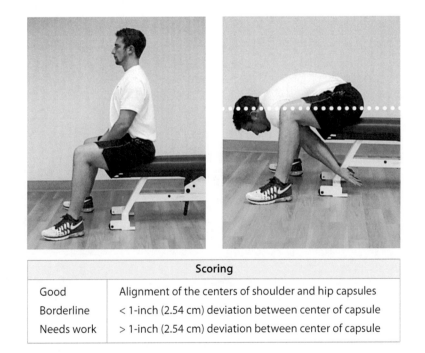

Scoring	
Good	Alignment of the centers of shoulder and hip capsules
Borderline	< 1-inch (2.54 cm) deviation between center of capsule
Needs work	> 1-inch (2.54 cm) deviation between center of capsule

Assessed Structures: _____

_____

Score _____

Notes: _____

3. **Unilateral Knee Flexion Test** *(page 342)*

Scoring
Good Heel touches glute without hip flexion
Borderline < 1 inch (2.54 cm) heel without hip flexion
Needs work > 1 inch (2.54 cm) with* or without hip flexion *indicates significant tightness in rectus femoris*

Assessed Structures: _____

_____

Left Score _____   Right Score _____

Notes: _____

4. **Active Knee Extension Test** *(page 343)*

Scoring	
Good	Lateral malleolus and the hip capsules
Borderline	< 3 inches (7.5 cm) deviation between center of capsule
Needs work	> 3 inches (7.5 cm) deviation between center of capsule

Assessed Structures: _____

_____

Left Score _____   Right Score _____

Notes: _____

Activity 2 **Mobility Assessment**

Activity Description

Mobility differs from flexibility by definition as well as performance implications. Flexibility is the attainable range of a single joint in a single plane while mobility reflects range and competence as multiple joints function together to create movement. The overhead (OH) squat assessment is commonly used to assess mobility as it requires interaction from joints of the shoulders, spine, hip, knees, and ankles. The interwoven fascia often experiences enhanced tension when multiple joints are employed simultaneously due to functional relationships, particularly among biarticular muscles.

Procedures

Have your volunteer subject perform an adequate warm-up prior to the OH assessment. Once the test subject is appropriately prepared, have them practice the test to confirm they understand the movement technique. This ensures a lack of proficiency doesn't provide a false positive result. Once proficient in the movement have the subject perform 12 repetitions of the OH squat. Evaluate 4 repetitions from the anterior (front) view, 4 from both lateral (side) views, and 4 from the posterior (rear) view. Report your findings at the end of each observation segment. Add detailed notes when reporting findings if there are bilateral inconsistencies or other observable findings which are relevant to the assessment. Finally, indicate the possible issues (tightness or weakness) which could be contributing to the movement inefficiency.

Front view notes:

_____

_____

Possible issues:

_____

_____

Side view notes:

_____

_____

Possible issues:

_____

_____

Rear view notes:

_____

_____

Possible issues:

_____

_____

Overhead Squat Test

☐ No Dysfunctions Noted

L	**Front View**	R
☐	Foot Turns Out	☐
☐	Knee Shifts In	☐
☐	Knee Shifts Out	☐

Side View

☐ Heels Lift

☐ Excessive Forward Lean

☐ Low Back Arch

☐ Low Back Rounds

☐ Arms Fall Forward

L	**Rear View**	R
☐	Foot Flattens	☐
☐	Asymmetrical Weight Shift	☐

Flexibility and Mobility Testing Lab Quiz

1. True or False? Bilateral assessments of flexibility are required as discrepancies often exist on opposite sides of the body.

    _____ a. True
    _____ b. False

2. The Apley back scratch tests assesses all of the following structures, except:

    _____ a. Subscapularis
    _____ b. Biceps
    _____ c. Anterior deltoid
    _____ d. Latissimus dorsi

3. Which of the following assessments examines ROM of the rectus femoris?

    _____ a. Trunk flexion test
    _____ b. Modified Thomas test
    _____ c. OH squat
    _____ d. Active knee extension test

4. Which of the following tests assess the ROM of the hamstrings?

    _____ a. Trunk extension test
    _____ b. Aply back scratch test
    _____ c. Trunk flexion test
    _____ d. Active knee extension test

5. Which of the following indicates a good score during the Modified Thomas test?

    _____ a. Straight leg contact with the bench
    _____ b. The knee is flexed all the way to the chest
    _____ c. The hamstring is 2-3 inches above the bench
    _____ d. The leg remains straight during the test

6. Which assessment examines abdominal (rectus abdominis) as well as hip flexor flexibility?

    _____ a. Trunk flexion test
    _____ b. Trunk extension test
    _____ c. Active knee extension test
    _____ d. None of the above assess these structures

7. Which of the following indicates a good score during the trunk flexion test?

    _____ a. The shoulders are 3-5 inches above the hip capsules
    _____ b. The shoulders are 3-5 inches below the hip capsules
    _____ c. The shoulders are aligned with the hip capsules
    _____ d. All are passing scores

8. True or False? Flexibility and mobility are synonymous terms and are associated with similar performance implications.

    _____ a. True
    _____ b. False

9. Which of the following issues is associated with excess hip adduction during the overhead squat test?

    _____ a. Weakness of the tibialis anterior
    _____ b. Weakness of the rectus abdominis
    _____ c. Weakness of the gluteal muscles
    _____ d. Weakness of the obliques

10. Which of the following issues is associated with the arms migrating forward in front of the body during the overhead squat test?

    _____ a. Iliopsoas weakness
    _____ b. Latissimus dorsi tightness
    _____ c. Hamstring weakness
    _____ d. Oblique tightness

◆ Anthropometric Measurements

This lab corresponds to the following text – Chapter 10: Pages 438-442, 445; Chapter 7: Pages 270-284

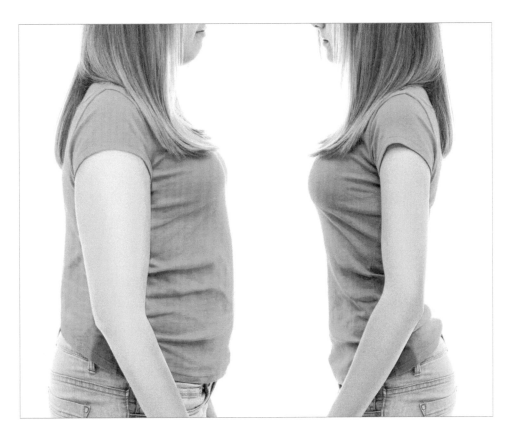

Activity 1 Calculating Body Mass Index (BMI)

Activity Description

Stature/weight indices compare the height of an individual to their weight to forecast risks for health problems based upon this relationship. Values are often compared to healthy weight ranges for specific populations based on all-cause morbidity and risks associated with deviations from identified healthy weight ranges. The predictions are based upon population norms and morbidity rates using height and weight ratios. They do not directly measure the amount of fat or lean mass on the body. The drawbacks to this are obvious. A person may have large amounts of lean mass and a relatively low quantity of body fat causing their weight to be dramatically higher than someone who has greater fat mass and less muscle. This would predict them as having an unhealthy weight and classify them in a higher-risk category even though they may actually be very healthy. That being said, larger people have greater risks for premature death compared to smaller people in general.

Body Mass Index (BMI) is the most common stature/weight index used to categorize people for risk of disease based on anthropometrics. The effectiveness of the BMI formula lies in its curvilinear relationship to the all-cause mortality ratio. The original formula uses a subject's mass (kg) divided by stature, height squared (m²). A newer formula using US customary units may be found to be easier for those less familiar with the metric system. Interpreting the BMI score as a measurement of body fat provides limited value, as proportional composition variables are not directly assessed. The norms for the BMI may imply that the higher the BMI of an individual, the greater the percentage of fat, but as stated earlier this may not always be the case – particularly for subjects with higher amounts of muscle mass. BMI's primary role is to serve as a clinical assessment tool to measure the appropriateness of a person's weight in relation to height. The lowest risk for disease is found within the BMI range of 20 to 25, with values exceeding 40 considered the highest risk. It has been suggested that the most desirable range is between 21.9 and 22.4 for males and between 21.3 and 22.1 for females. When BMI values surpass 27.8 for males and 27.3 for females the risk of hypertension, diabetes, and coronary artery disease increases. A person is considered overweight when their BMI is between 25 and 30, obese (class 1) when the value is greater than 30, and morbidly obese (class 2) when the value crosses 35. Note: Population norms for underweight, normal weight, overweight, and obese are based on BMI reporting, not on measurements of body composition.

Procedures

Complete the following activity using the procedures detailed below. You may use either the English or Metric formulas. Once a BMI value has been calculated for your test subject, reference the score using the tables in Chapter 10 to evaluate results.

Step 1 Measure and record the subject's weight:

_____ lb. _____ kg

Step 2 Measure and record the subject's height:

_____ inches _____ meters

Conversions
1 kg = 2.2 lb. 1 in = .0254 meters

Sample
5' 10" 150 lb. female
150 ÷ 2.2 = 68 kg
70 inches x .0254 = 1.778 m

Perform your conversion for the Metric formula below:

_____ lb. ÷ 2.2 = _____ kg

_____ inches x .0254 = _____ m

Step 3 Calculate your subject's BMI using one of the following formulas.

BMI Formulas

$BMI = \text{Weight in kilograms} \div \text{Height in meters}^2$

$BMI = (\text{Weight in pounds} \div \text{Height in inches}^2) \times 703$

Example One (English)
5'10" 150 lb. female
$BMI = \{150 \text{ lb.} \div (70 \text{ inches})^2\} \times 703$
$BMI = (150 \div 4900) \times 703$
$BMI = 0.0306 \times 703$
$BMI = 21.5$

Example Two (Metric)
5'10" 150 lbs. female
1.778 m 68 kg female
$BMI = 68 \div (1.788)^2$
$BMI = 68 \div 3.196$
$BMI = 21.3$

Perform your calculation below by selecting one of the two calculation methods:

BMI = { _____ lbs. ÷ (_____ inches)^2} × 703   BMI = _____ kg ÷ (_____ m)^2

BMI = (_____ lbs. ÷ _____) × 703   BMI = _____ kg ÷ _____

BMI = _____   BMI = _____

Classification of Weight by Body Mass Index (BMI), Waist Circumference, and Associated Disease Risks			
Category	**BMI (kg/m²)**	**DISEASE RISK RELATIVE TO NORMAL WEIGHT AND WAIST CIRCUMFERENCE**	
		Men <102 cm (40 in.) Women <88 cm (35 in.)	Men >102 cm (40 in.) Women >88 cm (35 in.)
Underweight	< 18.5	---	---
Normal	18.5 - 24.9	---	---
Overweight	25.0 - 29.9	*Increased*	*High*
Obese Class I	30.0 - 34.9	*High*	*Very high*
Obese Class II	35.0 - 39.9	*Very high*	*Very high*
Obese Class III	> 40.0	*Extremely high*	*Extremely high*

Relationship Between Body Mass Index and Percentage Body Fat									
Adult Males					**Adult Females**				
Age	**Increased Risk BMI < 18.5**	**Healthy BMI 18.5 - 24.9**	**Increased Risk BMI 25 - 29.9**	**High Risk BMI 30+**	**Age**	**Increased Risk BMI < 18.5**	**Healthy BMI 18.5 - 24.9**	**Increased Risk BMI 25 - 29.9**	**High Risk BMI 30+**
20 - 39	< 7.9%	8 - 19.9%	20 - 24.9%	> 25%	**20 - 39**	< 20.9%	21 - 28.9%	29 - 31.9%	> 32%
40 - 59	< 10.9%	11 - 21.9%	22 - 27.9%	> 28%	**40 - 59**	< 22.9%	23 - 29.9%	30 - 32.9%	> 33%
60 - 79	< 12.9%	13 - 24.9%	25 - 29.9%	> 30%	**60 - 79**	< 23.9%	24 - 31.9%	32 - 34.9%	> 35%

Activity 2 **Calculating Waist-to-Hip Ratio**

Activity Description

Shortly displaced by BMI and central girth measurements, waist-to-hip ratio has come back in vogue based on its predictability for sex-related health risk for cardiovascular disease and related disorders. It is well known that the risk for metabolic disease increases with central girth due to visceral fat storage, particularly when measures exceed 35 inches for females and 40 inches for males at the line of the umbilicus. But data provided by the hip measure improves prediction for certain diseases. And while it, like BMI, does not measure body fatness, the ratio can be measured more precisely than skinfolds and provides an index of (both) subcutaneous fat and visceral fat, whereas skinfold cannot. According to the World Health Organization, middle−aged men, assessed over a 12-year time period, showed that abdominal obesity (measured as waist−hip ratio) was associated with an increased risk of myocardial infarction, stroke and premature death, whereas these diseases were not associated with measures of generalized obesity such as BMI. In women, BMI was associated with increased risk of these diseases; however, waist-to-hip ratio appeared to be a stronger independent risk factor than BMI. These facts support the inclusion of waist-to-hip ratio in risk stratification for cardiovascular disease.

Equipment

- Measuring tape

Procedures

Step 1 *Identify the sites.*

Waist circumference should be measured across exposed skin, at the narrowest point between the lower margin of the least palpable rib and the top of the iliac crest.

Hip circumference should be measured over spandex or tight-fitting clothing, around the widest portion of the buttocks, with the tape parallel to the floor.

Make note of the clothing or take a picture to remind the subject to wear the same clothing for repeat measures.

Step 2 *Measure the sites.*

Have the subject stand with their feet close together, arms at the side and body weight evenly-distributed across the feet. The subject should be relaxed, and the measurements should be taken at the end of a normal expiration.

Each measurement is repeated twice; if the measurements are within 1 cm of one another, the average should be calculated. If the difference between the two measurements exceeds 1 cm, the two measurements should be repeated.

Step 3 *Record the sites and calculate the results.*

Waist Circumference _____ cm

Hip Circumference _____ cm

Waist measure _____ ÷ Hip measure _____ = _____ **W:H Ratio**

Step 4 *Assess risk.*

Risk for heart disease _____

Waist-to-Hip Ratio Norms for Men and Women								
Risk for Heart Disease	*Low*		*Moderate*		*High*		*Very High*	
Age (y)	Men	Women	Men	Women	Men	Women	Men	Women
20 - 29	<0.83	<0.71	0.83 - 0.88	0.71 - 0.77	0.89 - 0.94	0.78 - 0.82	>0.94	>0.82
30 - 39	<0.84	<0.72	0.84 - 0.91	0.72 - 0.78	0.92 - 0.96	0.79 - 0.84	>0.96	>0.84
40 - 49	<0.88	<0.73	0.88 - 0.95	0.73 - 0.79	0.96 - 1.00	0.80 - 0.87	>1.00	>0.87
50 - 59	<0.90	<0.74	0.90 - 0.96	0.74 - 0.81	0.97 - 1.02	0.82 - 0.88	>1.02	>0.88
60 - 69	<0.91	<0.76	0.91 - 0.98	0.76 - 0.83	0.99 - 1.03	0.84 - 0.90	>1.03	>0.90

Activity 3 The 2-3 Girth Estimation of Body Fat

Activity Description

Circumference estimation of body composition employs measurements of select locations to predict body fat. The methods are easy to perform and require minimal equipment. The assessment device is often no more than a common linen or plastic measuring tape. Often referred to as "girth measurements," they simply require the circumference measurement of designated sites of the body. The measured values are then charted, graphed, or equated based on the protocol being used. Depending upon the estimation model, girth measurements can predict body composition and help determine regional fat storage. The estimations are based on the positive linear relationship between the circumference values of anatomical areas and the amount of body fat a person carries.

Girth measurements are very practical assessment methods for fitness professionals and are considered psychologically-benign for most clients. When performed correctly with the appropriate prediction equation, they can have a standard estimate of error (SEE) of as little as 2.5% to 4%. They also provide useful information about fat distribution patterns as well as body fat changes during weight loss. Clients can see and understand the quantifiable differences found between measurements, which often serve as motivation even when bodyweight remains unchanged. Additionally, the methods are far more useful for measuring and predicting the body fat of obese individuals, as skinfold and other methods lose predictive value with higher levels of adipose tissue.

The 2-3 girth estimation of body fat is based on information gathered by the Naval Health Research Center (NHRC) and was developed from data collected on large samples of Navy men and women. The model has been found to have high correlations ($r = 0.85$ and 0.90) and reasonable standard errors ($SEE = 3.7\%$ and 2.7% among men and women, respectively) when compared to hydrostatic weighing. The 2-3 girth estimation is based on the linear relationship between circumference measurements and body fat. In the 2-3 girth method, the neck represents the reference value for lean body mass in both male and female models, whereas the abdominal and hip girths represent the fat factor for the prediction.

Equipment

- Measuring tape

Procedures

Follow the directions below to compute the 2-3 Girth estimation of body fat using a volunteer subject.

Step 1 ***Anthropometric data collection.*** Measure the appropriate anatomical locations of the subject and record the value in the space provided. All circumference measurements should be taken over the subject's skin where applicable. Tight fitting clothing or spandex should be worn when skin contact is not appropriate.

Men

- **Abdominal measurement** – circumference of the abdomen by aligning the tape so that it passes over the navel

- **Neck measurement** – circumference of the neck just inferior to the larynx (Adam's apple)

- Record your results.

Abdominal circumference	_____ in.
Neck circumference	_____ in.
Height	_____ in.

Women

- **Upper abdominal measurement** – circumference of the upper abdomen by aligning the tape so that it is between the distal aspect of the rib cage and the navel

- **Hip measurement** – circumference of the hip in the center of the gluteals at the level of the greater trochanter, or curvilinear apex, of the hip (widest point)

- **Neck measurement** – circumference of the neck just inferior to the larynx

- Record your results.

Upper abdominal circumference	_____ in.
Hip circumference	_____ in.
Neck circumference	_____ in.
Height	_____ in.

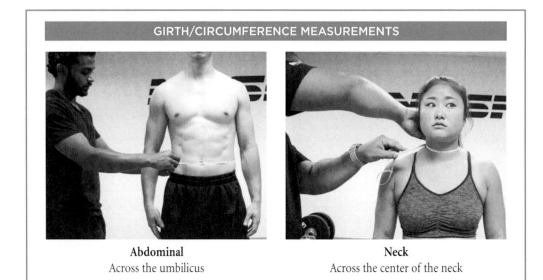

GIRTH/CIRCUMFERENCE MEASUREMENTS

Abdominal
Across the umbilicus

Neck
Across the center of the neck

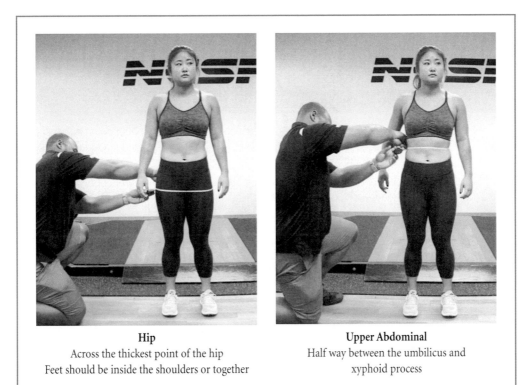

Hip
Across the thickest point of the hip
Feet should be inside the shoulders or together

Upper Abdominal
Half way between the umbilicus and
xyphoid process

Step 2 *Calculate the subject's derived circumference value.* The 2-3 girth model utilizes a derived circumference value to ascertain the subject's estimated body fat. From the data collected in Step 1, find the subject's derived circumference value by utilizing the following gender-specific equation.

Men: Abdominal – Neck = Circumference value

_____ – _____ = _____

Women: Upper abdominal + Hip – Neck = Circumference value

_____ + _____ – _____ = _____

Step 3 Calculate the derived body fat percentage using the following formulas or find the subject's estimated 2-3 girth percent body fat in your textbook.

To calculate a predicted body fat value (using inches):

Males: % body fat = {86.010 × (abdomen – neck)} – {70.041 × (height)} + 36.76

Females: % body fat = {163.205 × (waist + hip – neck)} – {97.684 × (height)} – 78.387

To find the estimated body fat using the graphs in your textbook:

Review the charts in Chapter 7 (page 275-284) which contain estimated body fat percentages according to the 2-3 girth model. To find your subject's estimated body fat you must first refer to the correct gender table (Table A for men and Table B for women). You must then match the subject's calculated circumference value from Step 2 with the subject's height in inches. The derived circumference values are located in the left-hand column and the height values are located across the top of the table.

Step 4 *Record data.* Record the subject's estimated 2-3 girth percent body fat value.

_____ Body fat percentage

Step 5 *Interpret the data.* Compare the subject's predicted body fat measurement with the following body fat percentage reference table.

Percent Fat in Men and Women		
Risk Category	**Men** *(% Body Fat)*	**Women** *(% Body Fat)*
Essential	3 - 5	11 - 14.9
Lean	6 - 10.9	15 - 18.9
Fitness	11 - 15.9	19 - 22.9
Healthy	16 - 19.9	23 - 26.9
Moderate Risk	20 - 24.9	27 - 31.9
High Risk	>25	>32

Male	<3%	5%	10%	15%	18%	22%	25%	30%
	Essential		*Lean*		*Early Risk*		*Obesity*	*Morbidly Obese*
Female	<11%	14%	16%	22%	26%	27%	32%	40%

Anthropometric Measurements Lab Quiz

1. What would be a client's disease risk classification if they have a BMI value of 32 with a waist circumference of 42 inches?

   ____ a. Increased
   ____ b. High
   ____ c. Very high
   ____ d. Extremely high

2. Which of the following does not measure fat mass within the body?

   ____ a. BMI
   ____ b. Waist-to-hip ratio
   ____ c. 2-3 girth measurements
   ____ d. All of the above

3. A 5' 11" 165 lb. male would have an estimated BMI of:

   ____ a. 18
   ____ b. 23
   ____ c. 25
   ____ d. 27

4. True or False? A client with a healthy level of body fat could be potentially scored as overweight according to a BMI value due to muscle mass.

   ____ a. True
   ____ b. False

5. Waist circumference indicates an increased risk for metabolic disease due to high _____ fat storage.

   ____ a. Subcutaneous
   ____ b. Visceral
   ____ c. Intramuscular
   ____ d. Lower body

6. The SEE for the 2-3 girth estimation of body fat can be as low as:

    _____ a. 2.5%
    _____ b. 4%
    _____ c. 5%
    _____ d. 10%

7. Which of the following is not measured among female clients when implementing the 2-3 girth estimation of body fat?

    _____ a. Upper abdominal circumference
    _____ b. Hip circumference
    _____ c. Upper arm circumference
    _____ d. Neck circumference

8. What body fat percentage among males is considered obese?

    _____ a. 20%
    _____ b. 25%
    _____ c. 32%
    _____ d. 40%

9. What body fat percentage among females is considered initial obesity?

    _____ a. 20%
    _____ b. 25%
    _____ c. 32%
    _____ d. 40%

10. What is the lowest percentage of body fat considered to meet essential needs among adult females?

    _____ a. 11%
    _____ b. 13%
    _____ c. 15%
    _____ d. 16%

◆ Body Composition and Metabolism

This lab corresponds to the following text – Chapter 7: Pages 284-288; Chapter 10: Pages 446-448, 450-451; Chapter 11: 466-469

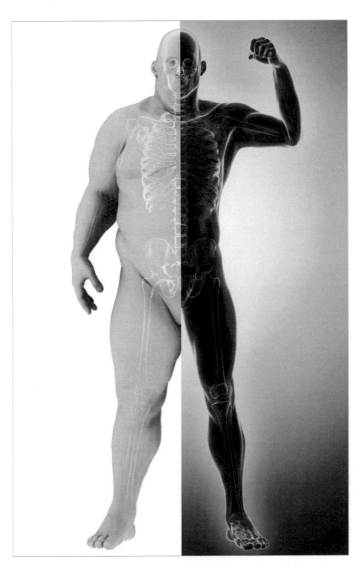

Activity 1 **Skinfold Estimation of Body Fat**

Activity Description

One of the most popular methods of assessing body fat employs the use of calipers to measure the thickness of skinfolds at select locations of the body. Subcutaneous fat is stored between the muscle and dermal layer of skin. It represents about 50%-70% of total fat stored in the body. The remaining fat surrounds visceral organs, is embedded within tissues in and around muscle, and circulates in the blood stream. Using regression equations, it is possible to predict the amount of fat mass a person has by measuring the thickness of skinfolds at specific sites.

There are several protocols to choose from when assessing an individual's body composition with skinfold calipers. The most common protocols use 2, 3, or 7 sites to obtain a predictive value for body fatness. Three site analysis has been shown to have a better predictive value than two sites; and using more than three sites has not conclusively shown to increase the accuracy of the assessment. Skinfold equations are typically within 3-4% of the value measured using underwater weighing. Assessing body composition by means of skinfold analysis requires a high degree of technical expertise and the technique of measuring skinfolds requires considerable practice; the technician must familiarize him or herself with the feel of the subcutaneous fold. This expertise is developed through continual practice on different subjects, as individual differences in the consistency of fat mass exist. Factors to consider include skinfold compressibility, skin tightness, edema, and variability in fat distribution. This supports the need for repeated practice before a technician becomes proficient at the technique and obviously suggests that the tester's expertise and adherence to the administration protocol affects the standard estimate of error (SEE) of this methodology.

Calibration and pincher selection will also affect the measurement. Pincher tension should be set at a constant 10 g/mm^2. Calipers that use manually-controlled pincher tension should be avoided for accurate assessment, as the actual tension cannot be reliably controlled. Additionally, the location of the fold measurement and speed of the reading can also affect accuracy. The fold should be measured in accordance with the description that follows to increase the accuracy of the measurement. A rapid reading is also important as fat is compressible and will "seep out" under the tension of the pinchers, therefore reducing the measure and subsequent prediction. Individuals that have excessive fat mass should be measured with girth measurements or similar replacement methodologies.

This lab will examine a 3-site measurement procedure formulated by Jackson and Pollock. The model measures the thickness of the subcutaneous fat in the chest, abdomen, and thigh of males, and triceps, suprailiac, and thigh of females. It is critical that the site of the skinfold measurement be accurately determined and marked before the assessment begins. This will increase the accuracy of the measurement. The site for measurement should be located and then marked with an erasable marker. This will help ensure that the calipers are placed precisely in the correct position each time the skinfold is measured. The exact location for the pinch and placement of the caliper will be explained in greater detail in the procedures section.

Procedures

Follow the description below to calculate the percent body fat using a sample subject and the 3-site skinfold method.

Step 1   *Locate the correct sex-specific anatomical location(s).* The chart and images on page 286 in Chapter 7 (or page 448 in Chapter 10) illustrate detailed descriptions of the male and female sites. Refer to these when locating the correct sex-specific skinfold locations. Once the site has been identified, mark the site with an erasable marker so that you can return to the exact location for subsequent measurements. This will also allow you to become more proficient at site identification and increase test reliability. **Note:** You may need to wipe the area dry of oils, sweat, or lotions before marking the site.

Jackson and Pollock Sex-Specific Skinfold Sites
- **Men**   Chest, Abdominal, Thigh
- **Women**   Triceps, Suprailiac, Thigh

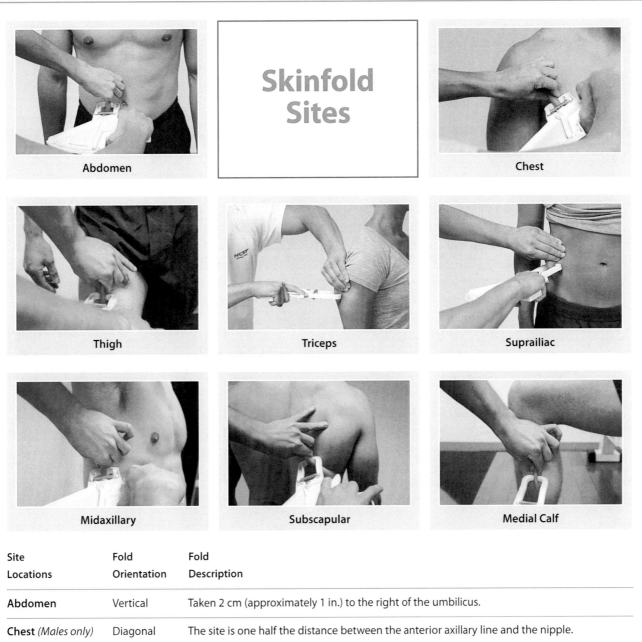

Skinfold Sites

Abdomen — Chest — Thigh — Triceps — Suprailiac — Midaxillary — Subscapular — Medial Calf

Site Locations	Fold Orientation	Fold Description
Abdomen	Vertical	Taken 2 cm (approximately 1 in.) to the right of the umbilicus.
Chest *(Males only)*	Diagonal	The site is one half the distance between the anterior axillary line and the nipple.
Thigh	Vertical	On the front of the thigh, midway between the hip (inguinal crease) and the superior aspect of the patella (kneecap).
Triceps	Vertical	Located halfway between the acromion process (shoulder) and the inferior part of the elbow on the rear mid line of the upper arm.
Suprailiac	Diagonal	Taken with the natural angle of the iliac crest at the anterior axillary line immediately superior to the iliac crest.
Midaxillary	Vertical	Fold is taken on the midaxillary line at the height of the xiphoid (end of sternum).
Subscapular	Diagonal	Just below the lowest angle of scapula, taken on a 45 degree angle toward the right side.
Medial Calf	Vertical	Seated with the right knee flexed and sole of the foot on the floor. The fold is taken on the medial side of the calf at its greatest circumference.

Step 2 *Hand placement.* Place the caliper in the right hand with the index finger on the trigger of the caliper. Slightly pronate the right hand so that the caliper can be easily read from above. Pronate the left hand to a point at which the thumb of the left hand is pointing downward. A simplified description is to have the tester place both arms out in front of him/her and rotate both arms inward so that both thumbs are pointing downward, with the caliper in the right hand. With the thumb and fore-finger facing downward, place the thumb and finger perpendicular to the marked site of the skinfold.

Step 3 *Pinching of skinfold.* Using a pinch width of approximately two inches, firmly pinch the skinfold between the thumb and first two fingers, lifting the subcutaneous fat and skin from the underlying muscle tissue.

Step 4 *Placement of calipers.* Once the tester has successfully separated the subcutaneous fat and skin from the underlying muscle belly, the calipers should be placed on the fold. The pinchers of the caliper should be placed across the long axis of the skinfold at the designated site. Using a 1 cm separation between the technician's fingers and the calipers should prevent the skinfold dimension from being affected by the pressure from the tester's fingers. The depth of caliper placement is about half the distance between the base of the normal skin perimeter and the top of the skinfold. Place the jaws of the calipers perpendicular to the skinfold site approximately 1 cm below the fingers. This will allow the caliper reading to be done approximately halfway between the bottom and top of the fold.

Step 5 *Reading of calipers.* Calipers have a compression tension of 10 g/mm^2. To get an accurate reading and prevent compression of the fat by the caliper, the tester must read the caliper to the closest half millimeter within 2 seconds of applying the caliper jaws to the fold. Measure each site and record the assessment values on the Data Recording Sheet. The measurements should be repeated two times allowing at least 15 seconds between subsequent measurements. If the measurements differ by more than 2 millimeters, a third measurement should be taken and an average of the three measurements used. In non-obese individuals, the skinfolds should not differ by more than two millimeters. The median values of the three trials are used for evaluation and prediction.

Step 6 *Record results.* Record the individual site measurements on the provided data recording form. The measurements will be used to compare future assessment results.

3-SITE SKINFOLD BODY COMPOSITION ESTIMATION DATA RECORDING FORM

Men:

Trial 1	Chest _____	Abdominal _____	Thigh _____
Trial 2	Chest _____	Abdominal _____	Thigh _____
Trial 3	Chest _____	Abdominal _____	Thigh _____
	Average _____	Average _____	Average _____

Sum of the three averages _____

Women:

Trial 1	Triceps _____	Suprailium _____	Thigh _____
Trial 2	Triceps _____	Suprailium _____	Thigh _____
Trial 3	Triceps _____	Suprailium _____	Thigh _____
	Average _____	Average _____	Average _____

Sum of the three averages _____

Step 7 *Computation of results.* Once the data has been recorded on the provided Data Recording Sheet, the tester should add the three skinfolds together to obtain the sum of skinfolds in millimeters. The sum of the skinfolds is then charted or used in a body density equation to determine the estimated body fat of the individual. The charts on pages 287-288 in Chapter 7 contain the estimated age-adjusted body composition computed by the Siri Equation. Find your subject's estimated body fat by referencing the sex-specific table and matching the sum of the skinfolds in the left-hand column with the subject's age on the top row.

Estimated Body Fat _____ %

Step 8 *Interpretation of results.* After the subject has been classified by an estimated value, the results can be used to establish goals and develop weight management strategies.

Percent Fat in Men and Women		
Risk Category	**Men** *(% Body Fat)*	**Women** *(% Body Fat)*
Essential	3 - 5	11 - 14.9
Lean	6 - 10.9	15 - 18.9
Fitness	11 - 15.9	19 - 22.9
Healthy	16 - 19.9	23 - 26.9
Moderate Risk	20 - 24.9	27 - 31.9
High Risk	>25	>32

Activity 2 Calculating Lean Mass & Target Body Weight

Activity Description

Differentiating the tissue compartments by mass is useful in determining the necessary changes for optimal health and goal setting for weight loss or gain. Using the percentage of body fat determined via body composition analysis, exercise professionals can identify the relative quantity of lean and fat mass on the body. These values can then be used to calculate target weight for appropriate adjustments in body composition.

Procedures

Following the instructions below, using the subject from the skinfold test, enter the appropriate data to calculate lean mass and target body weight. Use the examples provided for guidance.

Calculating Lean Mass	*Example*
Bodyweight × Body fat percentage = Fat mass weight	200 lb. male with 20% body fat
Bodyweight – Fat mass = Lean mass weight	20% ÷ 100 = 0.20
	200 lb. × 0.20 = 40 lb. Fat mass weight
	200 lb. – 40 lb. = 160 lb. Lean mass weight

Step 1   Enter estimated body fat   _____ %

Enter bodyweight   _____ lb.

Step 2   Enter the values from Step 1 into the formula.

Estimated body fat (_____ % ÷ 100) × bodyweight _____ lb. = _____ Fat mass

Step 3   Calculate lean mass by subtracting the fat mass, in pounds, from the total body weight.

Bodyweight _____ lb. – Fat mass _____ lb. = Lean mass _____ lb.

Step 4   Using the formula below, calculate the Target Body Weight based on the subject's desired percent body fat.

Lean Mass ÷ {1 – (NEW desired body fat percent ÷ 100)} = Target Body Weight

---

Example

200 lb. man 20% body fat

Lean Mass 160 lb.

New desired body fat 18%

160 lb. ÷ {1– (18% ÷ 100)} = Target Body Weight

160 lb. ÷ {1– (.18)} = Target Body Weight

160 lb. ÷ (.82) = 195 lb.

Current body weight 200 lbs. – Target body weight 195 lbs. = 5 lbs. weight loss

---

Step 5   Select a new Desired Body Fat   _____ %

Step 6   Enter the values from Step 1 and Step 2 into the formula below to calculate the Target Body Weight.

Hint: Do not convert the body fat percentage into a decimal before inserting the value.

Lean Mass _____ lbs. ÷ {1– (desired body fat percent _____ ÷ 100)} = Target Body Weight

Lean Mass _____ lbs. ÷ {1– (_____)} = Target Body Weight

Lean Mass _____ lbs. ÷ _____ = _____ Target Body Weight

Step 7   Subtract the Target Body Weight from the initial body weight to identify the weight loss goals.

Current body weight _____ – Target Body Weight _____ = Weight loss goal _____ lbs.

Once the initial short-term goal has been attained, an exercise professional should be able to re-compute the target body weight based on new desired body fat goals.

Step 8   In the following chart, calculate the desired weight for the subject as they lose body fat. Bodyweight should reflect a specific duration of time, reasonable fat loss goals, and account for the maintenance of lean mass.

Note: lean mass should NOT change during the calculation of predicted weight loss and body fat goals.

Starting Value	Goal #1	Goal #2	Goal #3
08/03/2019	09/07/2019	10/12/2019	11/15/2019
22%	*20%*	*18%*	*16%*
190 lb.	**185.25 lb.**	**180.7 lb.**	**176.4 lb.**

Starting Value	Goal #1	Goal #2	Goal #3
Date: _____	Date: _____	Date: _____	Date: _____
_____ %	_____ %	_____ %	_____ %
_____ lb.	_____ lb.	_____ lb.	_____ lb.

Activity 3 Individual Metabolic Needs Assessment

Activity Description

Metabolic assessment describes a variety of methods used to determine relevant information related to an individual's metabolic fitness and energy requirements. Health is dependent upon maintaining the sometimes-delicate balance between suitable body fuel to support energy needs and satisfying nutritional requirements to sustain proper biological function – without adding adipose tissue. Utilizing the proper assessment tools enable exercise professionals to identify possible areas that need to be addressed to help balance caloric requirements for varying clients' needs.

Metabolic rate represents the conversion of carbon-based energy to heat (calories) to facilitate the demands of the body's tissue. Resting metabolic rate (RMR) can be defined as the amount of energy needed to sustain the bodily functions under normal resting conditions. Each action that occurs within the body, whether physiological or biochemical, requires energy to support its activity. At rest, the brain and metabolic organs consume the majority of energy. This energy generates heat, which can be measured using direct calorimetry in a research laboratory. Researchers use this method to determine the specific energy costs of physiological activities. This form of assessment is very accurate but comes with a considerable monetary cost and large-scale delivery limitations. A less expensive version of calorimetry used to measure caloric expenditure is known as spirometry, or indirect calorimetry. This method analyzes oxygen utilization rather than heat production as the measurable criteria. Spirometry estimates the heat using the quantity of oxygen inhaled and carbon dioxide exhaled into a special breathing device. The caloric expenditure can be calculated using the respiratory exchange ratio (R) from the caloric equivalent of oxygen utilized.

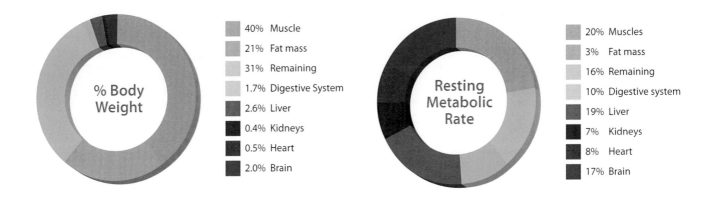

% Body Weight
- 40% Muscle
- 21% Fat mass
- 31% Remaining
- 1.7% Digestive System
- 2.6% Liver
- 0.4% Kidneys
- 0.5% Heart
- 2.0% Brain

Resting Metabolic Rate
- 20% Muscles
- 3% Fat mass
- 16% Remaining
- 10% Digestive system
- 19% Liver
- 7% Kidneys
- 8% Heart
- 17% Brain

Although these methods are accurate and provide valuable data for researchers in clinical lab settings, they have little relevance in the majority of personal training environments. Fortunately, there have been several additional methods developed to estimate metabolic rate. Using the scientific information gathered from researchers, we can now estimate metabolic rates using predictive formulas. Since RMR comprises approximately 60% to 70% of a person's daily caloric need, it is important for those engaging in weight loss, weight maintenance, or weight gain programs to know the approximate caloric intake needed for goal attainment. Through the estimation of RMR using the Harris-Benedict Formula or Cunningham Lean Mass Formula, a personal trainer can estimate the number of calories a person needs to sustain current body weight in a normal resting condition. The personal trainer can then assess the client's general activity level and make adjustments using the corresponding activity multiplier to calculate daily caloric need. This step is very important, as people do not regularly lay in bed all day.

Procedures

Using yourself or lab partner as a subject, follow the detailed steps below to calculate RMR using the RMR prediction equation. A 50-year-old, 215-pound, 6 foot tall, male subject is used as an example to assist you in the steps.

Harris-Benedict Equation

Males: $66 + (5 \times ht) + (13.8 \times wt) - (6.8 \times age)$

Females: $655 + (1.8 \times ht) + (9.6 \times wt) - (4.7 \times age)$

- RMR expressed in kilocalories per day
- ht (height) expressed in centimeters
- wt (weight) expressed in kilograms
- age expressed in years

Example Conversions:

215-pound male subject
215lb. ÷ 2.2 lb./kg = 97.7 kg

6-foot-tall subject
6 ft x 12 inches/ft = 72 inches
72 inches × 2.54 cm/in = 182.9 cm

Sample subject's RMR calculation

RMR = $66 + (5 \times ht) + (13.8 \times wt) - (6.8 \times age)$
RMR = $66 + (5 \times 182.9) + (13.8 \times 97.7) - (6.8 \times 50)$
RMR = 1,988 kcal per day

Step 1 Convert subject's body weight from pounds to kilograms

Test subject's weight _____ lb.

_____ lb. ÷ 2.2 lb./kg = _____ kg

Step 2 Convert height in inches to centimeters

Test subject's height _____ inches

_____ inches × 2.54 cm/in = _____ cm

Step 3   Calculate RMR in the spaces provided below by using your numbers from Steps 1 and 2 above. Be sure to use the correct sex formula.

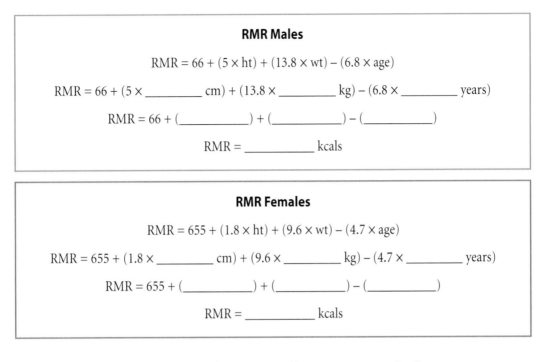

RMR Males

$$RMR = 66 + (5 \times ht) + (13.8 \times wt) - (6.8 \times age)$$

$$RMR = 66 + (5 \times \underline{\hspace{1.5cm}} cm) + (13.8 \times \underline{\hspace{1.5cm}} kg) - (6.8 \times \underline{\hspace{1.5cm}} years)$$

$$RMR = 66 + (\underline{\hspace{1.5cm}}) + (\underline{\hspace{1.5cm}}) - (\underline{\hspace{1.5cm}})$$

$$RMR = \underline{\hspace{1.5cm}} kcals$$

RMR Females

$$RMR = 655 + (1.8 \times ht) + (9.6 \times wt) - (4.7 \times age)$$

$$RMR = 655 + (1.8 \times \underline{\hspace{1.5cm}} cm) + (9.6 \times \underline{\hspace{1.5cm}} kg) - (4.7 \times \underline{\hspace{1.5cm}} years)$$

$$RMR = 655 + (\underline{\hspace{1.5cm}}) + (\underline{\hspace{1.5cm}}) - (\underline{\hspace{1.5cm}})$$

$$RMR = \underline{\hspace{1.5cm}} kcals$$

Estimated RMR for your test subject: _____ *(kcal)*

Lean Mass Estimation of RMR

The amount of lean mass a person carries influences RMR. It is widely-accepted that muscle is more metabolically-active than fat, even during resting conditions. This suggests that if two individuals weigh the same, the person with the higher amount of fat-free mass (FFM), or greater lean body weight (LBW), should have a higher RMR than the person with a higher amount of fat mass (FM). This further supports the need for a resistance training component in a fitness program aimed at weight loss.

Following the steps below, calculate the RMR value for your test subject. Use their body fat results from the previous equation to calculate RMR – now using the Cunningham Lean Mass Equation.

Cunningham Lean Mass Equation

Step 1   Determine lean mass value of subject using body composition analysis

Test subject's weight in pounds _____

Test subject's body fat percentage _____

Percent body fat × _____ weight in pounds = _____ fat mass

Weight in pounds – _____ fat mass = _____ fat-free mass

Step 2   Determine fat-free mass in kilograms

Fat-free mass in lb. _____ ÷ 2.2 = _____ fat-free mass in kilograms

Step 3 Calculate RMR from fat-free mass using the following formula

RMR (kcal/day) = 370 + (21.6 × fat-free mass in kg)

RMR (kcal/day) = 370 + (21.6 × _____ kg)

RMR (kcal/day) = 370 + (_____)

RMR = _____

Step 4 Compare the Cunningham Lean Mass RMR value to the Harris-Benedict RMR predication equation value.

Predicted RMR _____

Activity 4 **Estimating Daily Caloric Need**

Activity Description

A common error is using RMR and daily caloric need (DCN) synonymously. RMR is used to determine DCN, but only represents the number of calories a person expends at rest (recall the graphic from Activity 3). It is a reasonable assumption that a person will engage in some level of activity throughout the day, which may simply be activities of daily living (e.g., walking, climbing stairs, shopping, working), or may include participation in a formal exercise routine. Regardless, the number of calories expended each day must be accounted for when determining DCN. DCN represents the amount of calories needed to sustain current body weight while factoring in for average daily activities. It can be found by multiplying the RMR value by an Activity Factor. It is very important to choose an activity factor that best depicts the activity lifestyle of the client or an estimation error may occur. Most commonly, an overestimation of DCN occurs and leads to difficulty in weight loss goal attainment. The following tables provide information pertaining to the classification of a subject and their daily caloric need based on reported activity. This information is important to exercise professionals, as it will aid in establishing the proper nutritional program to meet a client's goals.

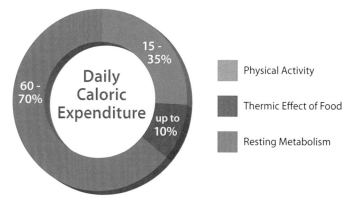

Procedures

Calculate your test subject's DCN by multiplying the RMR value from either the Harris-Benedict Equation or the Cunningham Lean Mass Equation by the correct corresponding Activity Multiplier.

RMR (kcal) × Activity Multiplier = Daily Caloric Need

RMR _____ kcal × Activity multiplier _____ = Daily Caloric Need _____ calories

Level of Intensity	Type of Activity	Activity Multiplier (x RMR)	Energy Expenditure (kcal • kg • day)
Very light	Seated and standing activities, professional jobs, laboratory work, typing, sewing, ironing, and cooking	1.3 Women 1.4 Men	30 31
Light	Walking on a level surface at 2.5 to 3 mph, garage work, electrical trades, carpentry, restaurant trades, house cleaning, child care, golf, sailing, and table tennis	1.5 Women 1.6 Men	35 38
Moderate	Walking 3.5 to 4 mph, landscaping, carrying loads, cycling, skiing, tennis, and dancing	1.6 Women 1.7 Men	37 41
Heavy	Walking with load uphill, tree work, heavy manual digging, basketball, climbing, football, and soccer	1.9 Women 2.1 Men	44 50
Vigorous	Athletes training in professional or world-class events	2.2 Women 2.4 Men	51 58

The more active an individual is, the higher the activity multiplier used will be. The activity multiplier can be adjusted to half-numbers (e.g., 1.45) to better account for those in between classifications. You can use the table to "classify" your client's fitness level; be aware though that it is more common for individuals to over-estimate their activity level. For a personal trainer working with a client who has weight loss as the primary goal, it is recommended to use the lowest reasonable activity multiplier to best meet the caloric restriction requirements needed for weight loss.

Body Composition Assessment and Metabolic/Energy Needs Lab Quiz

1. Subcutaneous fat represents _____ of total fat stored in the body.

    _____ a. 35-45%
    _____ b. 50-70%
    _____ c. 60-80%
    _____ d. About 95%

2. True or False? The seven-site skinfold estimation of body fat assessment has been found to have the greatest accuracy; nearly equal to underwater weighing.

    _____ a. True
    _____ b. False

3. Which of the following is not a female-specific skinfold site when using the Jackson-Pollack 3-site protocol?

    _____ a. Abdomen
    _____ b. Thigh
    _____ c. Triceps
    _____ d. Suprailiac

4. Which of the following is incorrect concerning skinfold assessments?

    _____ a. The folds must be held for 5 seconds to account for tissue compression
    _____ b. If measurements differ by more than 2 mm, a third measurement is needed
    _____ c. At least 15 seconds of rest should occur between measures at the same site
    _____ d. The calipers should have a compression tension of 10 g/mm^2

5. A male with 25% body fat would be considered _____ ?

    _____ a. Healthy
    _____ b. Obese
    _____ c. Lean
    _____ d. Underweight

6. What is the lean mass (estimated) of a 165 lb. female with 32% body fat?

    _____ a. 95 pounds
    _____ b. 112 pounds
    _____ c. 123 pounds
    _____ d. 140 pounds

7. Which of the following is needed to calculate daily caloric expenditure?

    _____ a. Physical activity
    _____ b. Resting metabolic rate (resting metabolism)
    _____ c. Thermic effect of food
    _____ d. All of the above

8. Which of the following contributes the most to one's resting metabolic rate?

    _____ a. Carbohydrate stores
    _____ b. Adipose tissue
    _____ c. Brain and metabolic organs
    _____ d. Lean mass

9. Which of the following can be used to estimate a client's resting metabolism?

    _____ a. Harris Benedict equation
    _____ b. Thermic Effect equation
    _____ c. Target Body Weight equation
    _____ d. None of the above

10. True or False? Resting metabolic rate and daily caloric need are synonymous.

    _____ a. True
    _____ b. False

Body Composition and Metabolism

◆ Nutritional Assessment

This lab corresponds to the following text – Chapter 8: Pages 348-351, 364-365, 371-379; Chapter 9: Pages 402-405

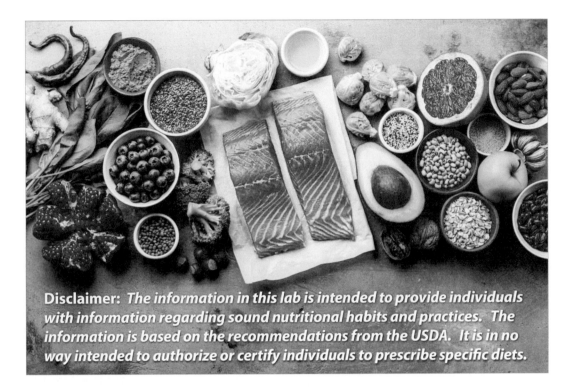

Disclaimer: *The information in this lab is intended to provide individuals with information regarding sound nutritional habits and practices. The information is based on the recommendations from the USDA. It is in no way intended to authorize or certify individuals to prescribe specific diets.*

Activity 1 **Reading a Food Label**

Activity Description

Decisions related to the improvement of dietary behaviors begins with an evaluation of intakes. The first step in the process is learning the difference between portions and serving sizes; an appropriate starting point is teaching the client how to properly read a food label. Although many exercise professionals will opt to utilize one of the many offered nutrition-analysis Apps, the information found on labels is relevant when educating clients as to what constitutes good and poor nutritional choices.

Many individuals are directed to follow the recommendations of the DRI-RDAs for energy nutrient consumption. The basic recommendation for caloric intake to reflect <30% of total calories from fat, 55%-60% from carbohydrates, and 10%-15% from protein is somewhat difficult to follow since computations are necessary to derive these values. Essentially, one must know their total caloric intake, the number of grams of each energy source consumed, and how to covert the numbers into a percentage of total calories. Fitness professionals using these recommendations must first understand how to calculate the percentages and then instruct their clients to be able to do the same. This process all starts with the ability to read a food label.

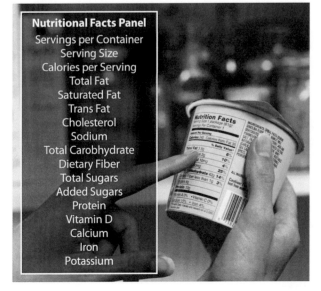

Nutritional Facts Panel
Servings per Container
Serving Size
Calories per Serving
Total Fat
Saturated Fat
Trans Fat
Cholesterol
Sodium
Total Carobhydrate
Dietary Fiber
Total Sugars
Added Sugars
Protein
Vitamin D
Calcium
Iron
Potassium

Procedures

The following food labels belong to a box of cereal, and a container of milk. For breakfast, a 174 lb. man consumed 2 cups of the cereal with 1 cup of milk. Review the labels and answer the questions that follow about the nutritional satisfaction of the meal for his daily requirements based on the food label content values for each nutrient *(Hint: percentage of calories is calculated by dividing the energy specific calories by total calories).*

Cereal Label	Milk Label

Nutrition Facts

8 servings per container

Serving size   **1 cup (55g)**

Amount per serving

Calories   **230**

	% Daily Value*
Total Fat 8g	**10%**
Saturated Fat 1g	**5%**
Trans Fat 0g	
Cholesterol 0mg	**0%**
Sodium 160mg	**7%**
Total Carbohydrate 37g	**13%**
Dietary Fiber 4g	**14%**
Total Sugars 12g	
Includes 10g Added Sugars	**20%**
Protein 3g	
Vitamin D 2mcg	10%
Calcium 260mg	20%
Iron 8mg	45%
Potassium 235mg	6%

* The % Daily Value (DV) tells you how much a nutrient in a serving of food contributes to a daily diet. 2,000 calories a day is used for general nutrition advice.

Nutrition Facts

About 8 servings per container

Serving size   **1 cup (240mL)**

Amount per serving

Calories   **90**

	% Daily Value*
Total Fat 0g	**0%**
Saturated Fat 0g	**0%**
Trans Fat 0g	
Polyunsaturated Fat 0g	
Monounsaturated Fat 0g	
Cholesterol <5mg	**1%**
Sodium 135mg	**6%**
Total Carbohydrate 13g	**5%**
Dietary Fiber 0g	**0%**
Total Sugars 12g	
Includes 0g Added Sugars	**0%**
Protein 8g	**16%**

Vitamin D 4.5mcg	25%	Calcium 300mg	25%
Iron 0mg	0%	Potassium 430mg	10%
Vitamin A 150mcg	15%	Riboflavin 0.4mg	30%
Vitamin B12 1.3mcg	50%	Phosphorus 250mg	20%

* The % Daily Value (DV) tells you how much a nutrient in a serving of food contributes to a daily diet. 2,000 calories a day is used for general nutrition advice.

Answer the following questions related to the food labels:

1. What is the total number of calories consumed by the individual?   _____ kcal

2. What percentage of the total calories consumed came from fat?   _____ %

3. What percentage of the total calories consumed came from carbohydrates?   _____ %

4. What percentage of the total calories came from sugars?   _____ %

5. How many grams of fiber did this person consume?   _____ g

6. What percentage of the total calories consumed came from protein?   _____ %

Activity 2 **Prediction of Energy Yielding Nutrient Requirements**

Activity Description

Physical activity is a primary determinant of daily energy requirement. Individual differences exist based on bodyweight, body composition, and the volume of physical activity performed routinely. Individuals who regularly engage in moderate-to-vigorous exercise and physical activity generally require more calories than comparably-sized individuals who are inactive. The determination of specific energy requirements is subject to several factors including the type of activity participated in and the volume and intensity employed on a weekly basis. The following activity identifies general recommendations related to these factors.

Procedures

Using the formulas below, calculate the energy intake requirements for each nutrient using yourself or a volunteer subject. The charts can be used to assist in identifying the specific requirements as they relate to individual size and physical activity status.

Carbohydrate Intake

Step 1 Convert bodyweight in pounds into bodyweight in kilograms.

Bodyweight _____ lb.

Bodyweight _____ lb. ÷ 2.2 = _____ kg

Step 2 Select a carbohydrate intake multiplier from the chart below based on your daily physical activity. If you fall in between whole values, you may use a decimal value (e.g., 4.5 g/kg of bodyweight).

Selected carbohydrate requirement _____ g/kg of bodyweight

The following example demonstrates the amount of carbohydrates needed for a 35 year old 5' 5" male, weighing 75 kg, who participates in regular, moderate exercise most days of the week.

Daily Caloric Intake		Population	Carbohydrate Requirements
Requirement	**2744 kcal**	Sedentary Individual	3-4 g/kg of body weight (BW)
Recommended CHO Intake	**60%**	Physically Active	4-5 g/kg of BW
Body weight in kilograms × selected active status		Moderate Exercise	5-6 g/kg of BW
Step 1: 75 kg × 5.5 g = 412 g		Vigorous Exercise	6-8 g/kg of BW
Step 2: 412 g × 4 kcal = 1648 kcal CHO			

Step 3 Multiply your weight in kilograms by your selected carbohydrate need.

Weight in kilograms _____ × selected carbohydrate need _____ g/kg = _____ carbohydrate intake requirement in grams

Carbohydrate intake requirement = _____ grams of CHO

Step 4   Multiply your carbohydrate intake requirement by 4 kcal/g carbohydrate to identify the predicted daily caloric intake requirement.

_____ grams of CHO × 4 kcal/g = _____ **Daily Carbohydrate Calories**

Protein Intake

Step 1   Convert bodyweight in pounds into bodyweight in kilograms.

Bodyweight _____ lb.

Bodyweight _____ lb. ÷ 2.2 = _____ kg

Step 2   Select a protein intake multiplier from the chart below based on your daily physical activity. If you fall in between whole values, you may use a decimal value (e.g., 1.45 g/kg of body weight).

Selected protein requirement _____ g/kg of bodyweight

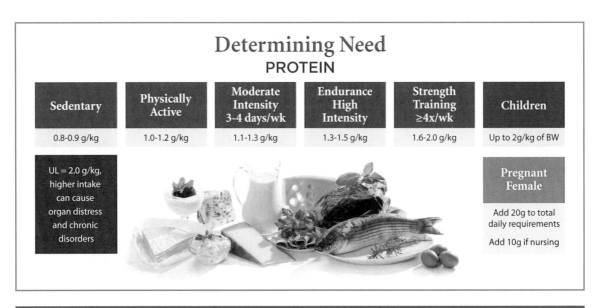

Sedentary	Physically Active	Moderate Intensity 3-4 days/wk	Endurance High Intensity	Strength Training ≥4x/wk	Children
0.8-0.9 g/kg	1.0-1.2 g/kg	1.1-1.3 g/kg	1.3-1.5 g/kg	1.6-2.0 g/kg	Up to 2g/kg of BW

UL = 2.0 g/kg, higher intake can cause organ distress and chronic disorders

Pregnant Female

Add 20g to total daily requirements

Add 10g if nursing

Determining Protein Needs

Body weight in lbs ÷ 2.2 lbs per kg = **Kilograms of body weight**

Kilograms of body weight × desired grams of protein per kilogram = **Daily protein requirement in grams**

Daily protein requirement in grams × 4 kcal per gram = **Total protein calorie requirement**

Example

220 lb Male
Population: Physically active

220 lbs ÷ 2.2 lbs per kg = 100 kg

100 kg × 1.1 grams per kg = 110 grams of protein

110 grams of protein × 4 kcal per gram = 440 kcal of protein

Step 3 Multiply your weight in kilograms by your selected protein need.

Weight in kilograms _____ × selected protein need _____ g/kg = _____ protein intake requirement in grams

Protein intake requirement = _____ grams of Protein

Step 4 Multiply your protein intake requirement by 4 kcal/g protein to identify the predicted daily caloric intake requirement.

_____ grams of Protein × 4 kcal/g = _____ **Daily Protein Calories**

Fat Intake

Step 1 Determine your total calories from Carbohydrates and Proteins (CHOPr) by entering your calculated carbohydrate and protein intake from above.

Carbohydrate intake _____ kcal + Protein intake _____ kcal = _____ CHOPr value

Step 2 Select a desired percentage of fat calories from the chart below.

Fat percentage _____ %

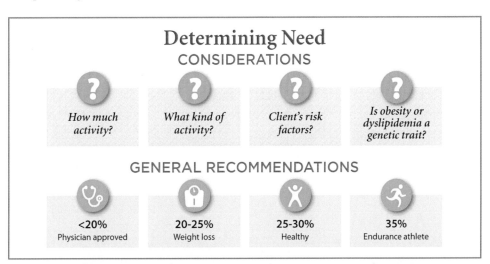

Determining Need
CONSIDERATIONS

| How much activity? | What kind of activity? | Client's risk factors? | Is obesity or dyslipidemia a genetic trait? |

GENERAL RECOMMENDATIONS

| <20% Physician approved | 20-25% Weight loss | 25-30% Healthy | 35% Endurance athlete |

Determining Fat Intake

Daily caloric need × recommended percentage of fat in the diet = **Calories of fat in diet**

Calories of fat in diet ÷ 9 cal per gram = **Grams of fat in the diet**

Grams of fat in the diet ÷ Kilograms of body weight = **Grams of fat per kg of bodyweight**

Example
220 lb Male
2744 Calorie per day diet
30% Recommended calories from fat

2744 cal × 30% = 823 calories of fat in diet

823 ÷ 9 cal per gram = 91 Grams of fat in the diet

91 ÷ 100 Kilogram of body weight = .91 Grams of fat per kg bodyweight

Step 3 Complete the formula below by entering your data.

Total calories = (CHOPr value _____ kcal) ÷ {1 – (desired percentage of fat _____ % ÷ 100)}

Total calories = _____

Step 4 Subtract the calculated carbohydrate and protein value (CHOPr value) from the total calories to identify the daily fat calories.

Total calories _____ – CHOPr value _____ = _____ **Daily Fat Calories**

Predicted daily caloric need based on the sum of the three calculations performed = _____ kcal

Nutritional Assessment Lab Quiz

1. It is recommended that an individual performing moderate exercise most days of the week should consume:

   ____ a. 3-4 g of carbohydrate per kg of body weight
   ____ b. 4-5 g of carbohydrate per kg of body weight
   ____ c. 5-6 g of carbohydrate per kg of body weight
   ____ d. 6-8 g of carbohydrate per kg of body weight

2. Strength training > 4 days per week requires what level of protein intake?

   ____ a. 1-1.3 g/kg of body weight
   ____ b. 1.3-1.5 g/kg of body weight
   ____ c. 1.6-2.0 g/kg of body weight
   ____ d. 3 g/kg of body weight

3. What is the lowest recommended level of fat intake per day without physician approval?

   ____ a. 10% of daily calories
   ____ b. 20% of daily calories
   ____ c. 30% of daily calories
   ____ d. 35% of daily calories

4. Which of the following may need fat intake above the daily recommendation for healthy adults?

   ____ a. Those trying to lose weight
   ____ b. Those engaging in heavy weight training
   ____ c. Those performing endurance sports
   ____ d. None of the above

5. Which nutrient should constitute the largest portion of daily calories among healthy adults performing regular exercise?

   ____ a. Carbohydrates
   ____ b. Fats
   ____ c. Proteins
   ____ d. All should be equal

6. Which of the following is not required on a standard food label?

    _____ a. Fiber content
    _____ b. Sugar content
    _____ c. Zinc content
    _____ d. Calcium content

The following questions are all related to the food label for a container of milk:

7. If a client consumed 2 cups in one sitting, how many grams of protein would be consumed?

    _____ a. 16 g
    _____ b. 24 g
    _____ c. 32 g
    _____ d. 48 g

8. If a client consumed 3 cups of milk in a day, how many calories from sugar would be consumed?

    _____ a. 120 kcals
    _____ b. 144 kcals
    _____ c. 158 kcals
    _____ d. 200 kcals

9. What percentage of total calories in each serving come from sugar?

    _____ a. 25%
    _____ b. 34%
    _____ c. 41%
    _____ d. 53%

Milk Label

Nutrition Facts

About 8 servings per container

Serving size   1 cup (240mL)

Amount per serving

Calories   **90**

	% Daily Value*
Total Fat 0g	0%
Saturated Fat 0g	0%
Trans Fat 0g	
Polyunsaturated Fat 0g	
Monounsaturated Fat 0g	
Cholesterol <5mg	1%
Sodium 135mg	6%
Total Carbohydrate 13g	5%
Dietary Fiber 0g	0%
Total Sugars 12g	
Includes 0g Added Sugars	0%
Protein 8g	16%

Vitamin D 4.5mcg	25%	Calcium 300mg	25%
Iron 0mg	0%	Potassium 430mg	10%
Vitamin A 150mcg	15%	Riboflavin 0.4mg	30%
Vitamin B12 1.3mcg	50%	Phosphorus 250mg	20%

* The % Daily Value (DV) tells you how much a nutrient in a serving of food contributes to a daily diet. 2,000 calories a day is used for general nutrition advice.

10. How many servings would need to be consumed to obtain 100% of one's daily calcium needs?

    _____ a. 2
    _____ b. 3
    _____ c. 4
    _____ d. 6

◆ Exercise Programming

This lab corresponds to the following text – Chapter 7: Page 321; Chapter 12: Pages 482, 489-503; Chapter 13: Pages 531-538

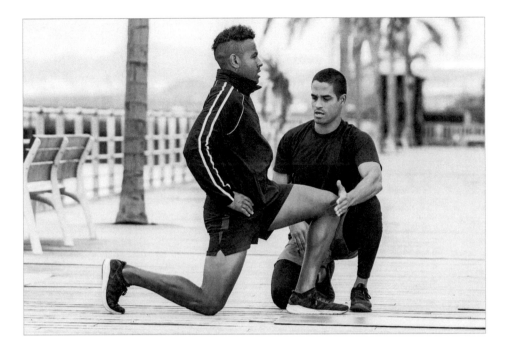

Activity 1 Exercise Principles and Components of Programming

Activity Description

In order to properly prescribe exercises and create effective programs, the principles of exercise must be appropriately applied within training activities. The correct application of these principles creates the adaptation stress to optimize programmatic effectiveness and reduces the risk of injury.

Exercise Order

Although there are countless training activities and techniques, there are some simple rules that can be applied to help formulate the exercise prescription as it relates to exercise order. It is important to understand that these guidelines are general in scope and should not be viewed as the end-all to resistance training programming, as individual factors may warrant additional consideration or adjustments. The systems of the body provide the key insight as to what goes where in a training program and within an individual workout. Starting with the metabolic pathways, training always follows the energy systems from stored ATP to aerobic metabolism. Consider the following:

Energy system	Contraction type	Force output	Exercise example
Creatine Phosphate (0-10 sec)	Plyometric/Ballistic	High	Olympic lifts
Creatine Phosphate (10-15 sec)	Dynamic	High	Squat/Deadlift
Creatine-Glycolytic (15-20 sec)	Ballistic	High	Anaerobic power step
Glycolytic (20-40 sec)	Dynamic	Moderate-high	Walking lunges
Glycolytic (40-90 sec)	Dynamic/Ballistic	Moderate	200-400 m run
Aerobic (>90 sec)	Ballistic	Low	Cycling/Jogging

Exercise order is also a factor of the speed of the movement, total muscle mass involved, difficulty of the task, interaction of stabilizers, and number of joints involved. When following the systems-approach, the order is based on the contribution and interaction between systems involved in movement.

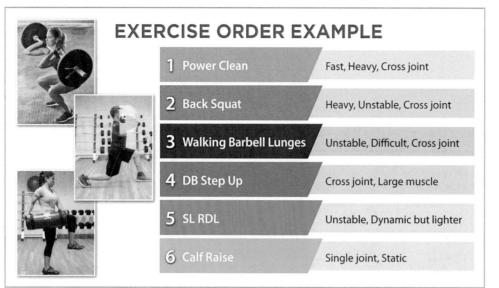

EXERCISE ORDER EXAMPLE

1	Power Clean	Fast, Heavy, Cross joint
2	Back Squat	Heavy, Unstable, Cross joint
3	Walking Barbell Lunges	Unstable, Difficult, Cross joint
4	DB Step Up	Cross joint, Large muscle
5	SL RDL	Unstable, Dynamic but lighter
6	Calf Raise	Single joint, Static

- High intensity to low intensity
- Fast movements to slow movements
- Large muscle groups to small muscle groups
- Complex movements (multi-joint) to simple movements (single joint)
- High skill level to low skill level or unstable to stable
- Multiplane movements to single plane movements

Note: If deficiencies exist, they should be addressed as a priority in the exercise prescription and may precede the above order recommendations. Additionally, programming should reflect the needs analysis, which is based on exercise assessment results and goals.

Procedures

Proper exercise order is a relevant part of the total exercise prescription. The following groups of exercises are not in proper order. Place them in the appropriate order, keeping in mind the standard principles of order. Assume each exercise is performed to volitional failure using 8-10 repetitions (~75-80% 1RM).

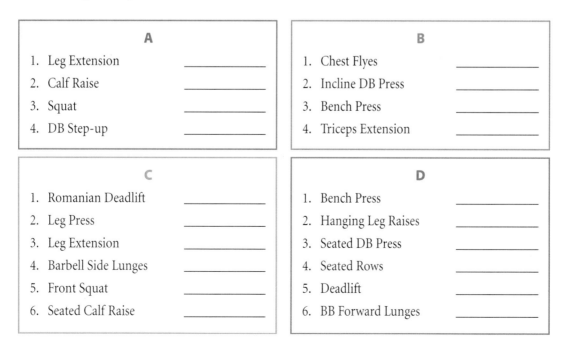

A

1. Leg Extension _____
2. Calf Raise _____
3. Squat _____
4. DB Step-up _____

B

1. Chest Flyes _____
2. Incline DB Press _____
3. Bench Press _____
4. Triceps Extension _____

C

1. Romanian Deadlift _____
2. Leg Press _____
3. Leg Extension _____
4. Barbell Side Lunges _____
5. Front Squat _____
6. Seated Calf Raise _____

D

1. Bench Press _____
2. Hanging Leg Raises _____
3. Seated DB Press _____
4. Seated Rows _____
5. Deadlift _____
6. BB Forward Lunges _____

Rest Intervals

Procedures

Rest intervals are necessary for the rephosphorylation of ATP, the management of hydrogen ions, as well as indicating the hormonal response to the stress of exercise. Specific rest intervals can be used to optimize the adaptation process and must be considered for the proper implementation of exercise programs. Incorrect rest intervals change the perception of stress and modify the outcome. Personal trainers must identify the rest interval required for the desired outcome and understand the relationship between the energy system and the work-to-rest ratio. Complete the following table by entering the correct information for the specific goal or outcome.

Intended Outcome	Activity	Energy System	Rest Interval
Example: Aerobic conditioning	Cardio-circuit	Aerobic/glycolytic	Transitional rest <15 sec
Hypertrophy	Bicep curls 10 reps		
Strength	Back squats 5 reps		
Anaerobic endurance	Push-ups 20 reps		
Anaerobic power	High box jumps 4 reps		

Exercise Principle Applications

Procedures

The key principles of exercise include specificity, overload, and progression. In many cases, the latter two combine to form progressive overload. Each holds merit in the design of an exercise program. Review the following definitions and complete the activity questions that follow.

Fundamental Principles of Exercise:		
Specificity	**Overload**	**Progression**
For a desired adaptation to occur in the body, stress must be appropriately and specifically applied	A training stress that challenges a physiological system above the level to which it is accustomed	Stress applied must continually be perceived as new for any physiological system to adjust

Principle of Specificity

As the name implies, specificity refers to the goal-oriented outcome of a particular action or activity. In the case of resistance training, the training effect is specific to the physiological systems used and method of overload applied. Programs should have goal-oriented outcomes and the exercises selected must be specific to the attainment of the desired goals. For example, a person looking to increase power output would not gain performance benefits by performing weight training in a slow, controlled manner. Likewise, muscle size and strength are specific to the muscle groups and the motor units activated and stressed. The exercise, intensity, and volume must be specific to the desired outcome. Training specificity is the key to eliciting the proper effects of exercise. Review the following training goals and place the letter that corresponds to the appropriate exercise selection identified as specific to the intended goal. Some of the activities will not be used to attend to the goals, therefore pick the best selection of the activities listed.

Goal	Activity
_____ Reduce upper arm fat	a. Supine triceps extension
_____ Increase core stabilization	b. Romanian deadlift
_____ Increase hamstring strength	c. Chair stands
_____ Increase glute range of motion	d. Bulgarian (Single-leg) squat
_____ Frontal plane, closed-chain movement proficiency	e. OH Squat
_____ Power exercise for an older adult	f. High box step-up
_____ Dynamic flexibility for the hip flexor	g. 20 minute interval training
	h. Lateral lunge
	i. Bench press

Principle of Overload

Overload is defined as a stress level beyond that to which the body is presently accustomed. It is the sole reason that the body adapts to exercise. Adaptations will occur if physiological systems experience new perceived stress. Once the stress no longer exceeds the current level that the body is accustomed to, adaptations will subside. This explains why people may workout for a period of time, and not make any new gains from the previous training period. If the body does not experience any new stress greater than that by which it is normally accustomed, no new adaptations will occur.

Procedures

Identifying the proper quantity of overload is necessary for progressive adaptation responses. Insufficient stress or excessive stress will not create the desired outcome from training. Exercise professionals must recognize the proper degree of overload for their clients while staying within the appropriate confines of ability and exercise tolerance.

> ***Sample Subject:*** A client was able to perform a 200 lb. bench press for 5 repetitions. Complete the calculations to determine the loads to support the overload demands.

Step 1 Calculate the 1RM from a chosen multi-rep test 1RM (see full protocol in Muscular Fitness Testing Lab if not yet performed) = **weight used × {(Reps performed x 0.03) +1}**

$$1RM = \underline{\hspace{2in}}$$

> **Sample:** 1RM = 200 lb. × {(5 x 0.03) +1}
> 1RM = 200 lb. × 1.15
> 1RM = 230 lb.

Step 2 Determine the amount of weight to be lifted during the exercise based on desired repetitions.

How much weight would be used? **Exercise weight = 1RM ÷ {(Desired reps x 0.03) +1}**

$$Exercise\ weight = \underline{\hspace{2in}}$$

> **Sample:** Subject will perform 10 repetitions
>
> Exercise weight = 230 ÷ {(10 x 0.03) +1}
>
> Exercise weight = 230 ÷ 1.3
>
> Exercise weight = 177 lb. (round down to 175 lb.)

Step 3 Calculate the level of training capacity.

Exercise weight ÷ 1RM = Training intensity percentage

Training intensity percentage × {(.03 x rep range) + 1} = Training capacity

Training capacity = _____

> **Sample:** 175 lb ÷ 230 = 76% 1RM
>
> Training capacity = 76% 1RM × {(.03 × 10) + 1}
>
> Training capacity = 76% × 1.3
>
> Training capacity = 98.8%

Step 4 Perform the exercise using the repetitions with the defined weight for 3 sets to achieve overload.

Principle of Progression

The principle of progression is quite basic, but many programs fail because it is not effectively incorporated into the exercise design. Progression is simply the planned application of the overload principle. Applying progressive overload throughout a training cycle allows the body to adapt to the stress and improve. The improvement may be neural, biochemical, structural, or all three. For continual improvement over a time segment, the overload must be thoughtfully considered. A general recommendation is to increase the overload by 2.5-5% once a repeated performance in two consecutive training sessions of the previous goal weight or stress is attained.

Procedures

Regardless of the type of training program you wish to prescribe, you must choose appropriate starting points and exercise program progressions for the client. The selection of appropriate starting points and progressions will be based primarily on assessments, observations, and client feedback. Having a thorough understanding of the specific demands of a multitude of training techniques will enable you to adjust a client's routine to better accommodate individual abilities and the rate of physiological adaptations. In general, adaptations are based on the stress and therefore the stress should change to reflect the goal. Consider the following progressions across a training cycle in the sample; complete the table using the same concept.

Technique	Load	Challenge	Speed
Example: Lunge	Barbell Lunge	Walking Lunge	Jump Lunges
Seated DB press			
DB squat to press			
Pull-up			
Bench push-up			
Box step-up			

Activity 2 **Training Systems**

Activity Description

Exercise prescription for personal training clients rely on creative, but logical strategies to apply adequate training stresses in limited periods of time. The application of training systems allows for different types of program dynamics aimed at a variety of adaptational responses in a single exercise regimen. Utilizing the systems properly and in conjunction with exercise principles allows for more efficient goal attainment than traditional set-rep schemes.

Procedures

Training principles can be further employed using anaerobic and aerobic training systems. The systems allow for the application of progressive overload specific to the desired outcome. Complete the table by identifying the type of system utilized and the specific outcome that it is designed to meet.

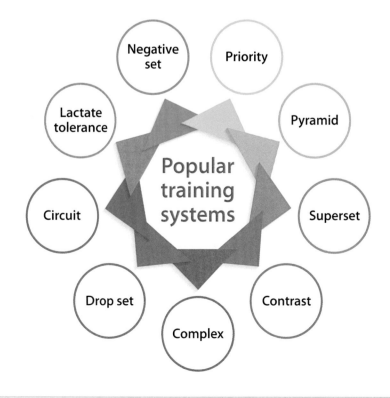

Training System	Activity	Rest Interval	Goal of Training
Example: Superset	10 repetitions of barbell supine triceps extension followed by close grip bench for repetitions to failure	30-60 seconds	Hypertrophy
	5 repetitions of squats immediately followed by 6 squat jumps	2 minutes following system	
	Seven exercises performed sequentially	Transitional period	
	DB chest press immediately followed by DB lunge immediately followed by stability ball crunch (each for 12 reps)	60-90 seconds	
	Leg press 10 reps using 75% 1RM – full rest interval 8 reps using 80% 1RM – full rest interval 6 reps using 85% 1RM	90-120 seconds	

Activity 3 **Exercise Selection**

Procedures

Proper exercise selection, particularly during the initial program design, is an important part of the total exercise prescription. The following activity requires you to review the sample case study and decide whether the listed exercise represents an appropriate selection for the initial training prescription. After deciding to include the exercise or not, defend the rationale for your answer in the space provided. You may modify the exercise in your justification to include it in the program.

Sample Subject

Bob is a 49-year-old sedentary male. He is six feet tall and weighs 200 lbs. with a body composition of 20%. He complains of intermittent low back pain and has hypertension, but has been cleared for exercise. His fitness evaluation scores are as follows:

Push-up:	5
Ab-curl:	10 – difficulty maintaining posterior pelvic tilt (feet lift)
Squat:	Cannot perform technique properly (heels cannot stay down)
VO$_2$max:	29 ml/kg/min
Flexibility:	Tight hamstrings, tight glutes, tight upper back, poor shoulder flexion and rotation
Movement efficiency:	Has average movement skills
Goal:	Overall improvement in health and fitness

Exercise	Yes/No	Why? – Defend your Answer
Back squat with bar		
Walking lunges with dumbbells		
Leg press		
RDL with bar		
Leg extension		
Lateral lunge		
Supine triceps extension		
Seated shoulder press with bar		
Seated row		
DB side raise		
Deadlift		
Back extensions		
Push-ups from floor		

Activity 4 **Exercise Prescription**

Procedures

Exercise prescriptions require many considerations to be properly formulated. Depending on the individual's goals and fitness needs, the prescription should reflect their current fitness status, abilities, and availability of time. Personal training for results can be difficult with all the needs most clients have and the limited amount of time available to fit it all in. The following activity requires you to create a prescription overview that identifies when each muscle group will be trained (frequency).

Sample Subject

The subject is a 33-year-old female. She is 5'7" tall and weighs 140 lbs. She is interested in improving her fitness level and toning her muscles. She can workout three days a week for an hour on Monday, Tuesday, and Thursday, and is willing to perform aerobic activity without your supervision. Using her data, create a general model for her exercise program by placing the muscle groups in the table to create her basic exercise model; muscle groups may be used more than once. Then, specify an exercise that trains each muscle group.

Body composition:	28%	**Abdominal curl-up:**	20
Modified push-up:	9	**Anaerobic step 1 min:**	307 watts (50th percentile)
Modified pull-up:	7		

The minimum training parameter for each muscle group is to be trained at least twice per week. Make appropriate considerations for recovery (rest).

Chest	Biceps	Shoulders
Quadriceps	Triceps	Hamstrings
Low Back	Aerobic activity	Back *(lats, rhomboids, trapezius)*
Calves	Glutes	Abdominals
Adductors	Obliques	

Sunday	Monday	Tuesday	Wednesday

Thursday	Friday	Saturday

Activity 5 **Creating a Circuit Training Program**

Procedures

Circuit training is an excellent method for eliciting several health responses using resistance training in a relatively short period of time. It can provide a great avenue for caloric expenditure, cardiovascular and strength benefits, as well as increasing volume with limited time availability. Create a circuit training program for the following individual.

Age:	42
Gender:	Male
Body Composition:	23%
Activity Level:	Previously sedentary
Goal:	Improved health
Time Constraints:	Subject has 30 minutes 3 days/week

Intensity: _____% (1RM)

Frequency: _____ days/week

Work Interval: _____ (sec)

Rest Interval: _____ (sec)

No. of Stations: _____

Time for Completion: _____ (1 Circuit)

No. of Circuits/Session: _____

1. _____

2. _____

3. _____

4. _____

5. _____

6. _____

7. _____

8. _____

9. _____

10. _____

11. _____

12. _____

Procedures

For the same individual, provide a single-day excerpt of a three-day (Mon, Wed, Fri) strength training program. The subject has engaged in your circuit program for four weeks and has been re-assessed for strength. His re-test values indicate he is ready to advance to more challenging activities. Based on his new goal of added strength, proper progression dictates allowing him to participate in a more comprehensive strength program. Fill in the boxes on the following table to create his single-day workout. Assume a warm-up and cool down are already included.

Exercise	Sets/Reps	Intensity	Rest Period

Exercise Programming Lab Quiz

1. Performing four repetitions of the modified deadlift would fall within which metabolic pathway:

   _____ a. Aerobic
   _____ b. Glycolysis
   _____ c. Creatine phosphate
   _____ d. Resting ATP

2. Which of the following would be performed first within an exercise session?

   _____ a. Seated calf raise
   _____ b. Military press
   _____ c. Bodyweight walking lunges
   _____ d. Front squat

3. What would be the most appropriate rest period for a client performing 12 reps of a triceps cable push-down exercise?

   _____ a. 30-45 sec
   _____ b. 60-90 sec
   _____ c. 90-120 sec
   _____ d. Transitional rest

4. Longer rest intervals are necessary for the resynthesis of _____ during workouts for muscle strength.

   _____ a. Lactate
   _____ b. Hydrogen ions
   _____ c. Aerobic enzymes
   _____ d. Creatine phosphate

5. Which exercise principle states that a training stress must challenge a physiological system above the level it is accustomed for adaptations to occur?

   _____ a. Principle of oxidation
   _____ b. Principle of specificity
   _____ c. Principle of overload
   _____ d. Principle of progression

6. Which of the following would be the most appropriate choice for helping a client who has weak hamstrings?

_____ a. Leg press
_____ b. Overhead squat
_____ c. Romanian deadlift
_____ d. Front squat

7. A general recommendation is to increase applications of overload by _____ per week.

_____ a. 0.5-1.5%
_____ b. 2.5-5%
_____ c. 3-7%
_____ d. 5-10%

8. Which of the following training systems will help improve power via fast twitch fiber recruitment?

_____ a. Negative set
_____ b. Superset
_____ c. Drop set
_____ d. Contrast set

9. Which of the following can be obtained via the use of circuits?

_____ a. High caloric expenditure
_____ b. Increased anaerobic endurance
_____ c. Improved dynamic flexibility
_____ d. All of the above

10. Which of the following supersets would be the best choice for a client working on hypertrophy?

_____ a. Deadlift followed by MB chest pass
_____ b. DB press followed by DB lateral raises
_____ c. Leg curls followed by bicep curls
_____ d. Seated row followed by push-ups

Exercise Programming

◆ Aerobic Exercise Prescription, Caloric Expenditure, and MET Intensity

This lab corresponds to the following text – Chapter 14: Pages 558-564, 568-572

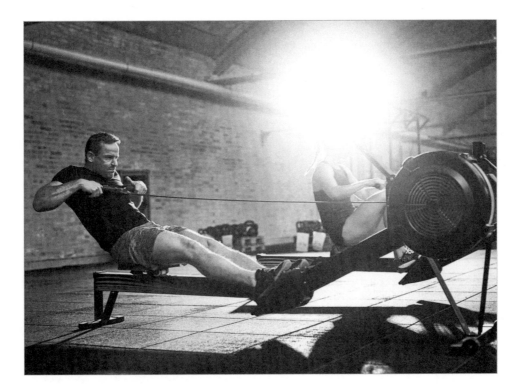

Activity 1 Calculating Maximum Heart Rate and Aerobic Training Intensities

Activity Description

Consistent aerobic training can increase aerobic capacity (VO_2) by up to 15%-30%. This value may increase even more with continued training at progressively higher intensities. The specific physiological adaptations that occur in response to regular aerobic training include: enhanced aerobic enzyme activity, which facilitates more efficient carbohydrate and lipid breakdown; increased muscle fiber capillary density, which allows for increased oxygen to the working muscles and increased by-product waste removal; and increased mitochondrial density, contributing to greater oxygen utilization. At the same time, the heart responds by increasing contractile force and stroke volume which in turn decreases resting and exercise heart rate responses at the same relative intensities. Together, cardiac and skeletal muscle adaptations increase the body's capacity to circulate, deliver, and utilize oxygen, which translates to increases in VO_2max and a more efficient cardiorespiratory system.

The term "Aerobic Intensity" refers to the amount of physical exertion the body experiences when performing an activity or exercise. Aerobic exercise intensity reflects the speed of the movement, or resistance to the movement, and is usually physiologically quantified by the subject's heart rate response at a given workload. For maximal gains in cardiorespiratory fitness to take place, ideal training intensity zones have been established which utilize specific heart rate responses based on workloads. The two most commonly accepted methods of calculating training intensity zones are based on heart rate and utilize either the Heart Rate Max Formula or Heart Rate Reserve Formula (HRR). The formulas use a predicted maximum heart rate based on age. **Note:** the traditional Heart Rate Max Formula may be off as much as 10-24 beats/min in 32% of the population (Standard Deviation = at least 10-12 bpm based on the bell curve theory).

Procedures

This activity requires the calculation of a subject's training intensities using two different methods (you have the option of calculating your own or a subject).

Step 1   Assess the resting heart rate and record base information:

Resting Heart Rate of subject _____ beats/min

Age of subject _____

Step 2   Calculate Maximum Heart Rate for your subject using the indirect method.

220 – Age = predicted Max Heart Rate

220 – _____ subject's age = _____ predicted Max Heart Rate

Record subject's predicted Max Heart Rate value: _____ beats/min

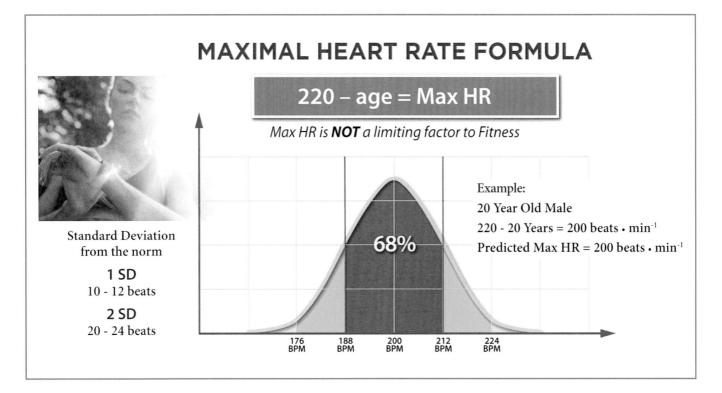

Step 3   Calculate subject's Target Heart Rate Zone using the Max Heart Rate Method and the recommended (75%-90%) training intensities.

Sample Subject:	*Find the recommended training zones using the Max Heart Rate Method and corresponding intensity ranges.*
45-year old male with a resting heart rate of 77 beats/min	175 beats/min × **.75** = 130 beats/min *(Low end)*
Find the predicted max heart rate.	175 beats/min × **.90** = 158 beats/min *(High end)*
220 – 45 = 175 beats/min	**Target Heart Rate Zone** = 130 beats/min to 158 beats/min

Enter the predicted max heart rate of the subject from Step 2 and calculate the Target Heart Zone using the intensities provided.

_____ Max HR × (.75) = _____ (L)

_____ Max HR × (.90) = _____ (H)

Record the low end and high end of the training zone.

Target Heart Rate Zone = (L) _____ to (H) _____ beats/min

Step 4 Calculate the subject's Target Heart Rate Zone using the Heart Rate Reserve (HRR) Method and recommended corresponding training intensities (60%-80%).

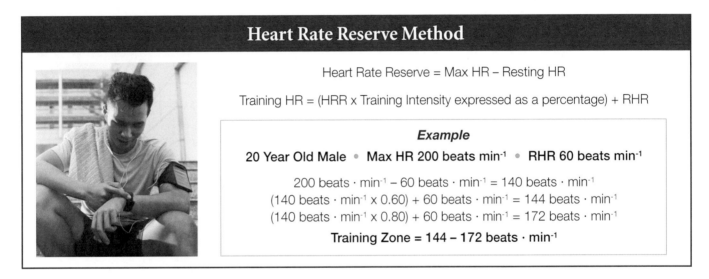

Heart Rate Reserve Method

Heart Rate Reserve = Max HR – Resting HR

Training HR = (HRR x Training Intensity expressed as a percentage) + RHR

Example
20 Year Old Male • Max HR 200 beats min⁻¹ • RHR 60 beats min⁻¹

200 beats · min⁻¹ – 60 beats · min⁻¹ = 140 beats · min⁻¹
(140 beats · min⁻¹ x 0.60) + 60 beats · min⁻¹ = 144 beats · min⁻¹
(140 beats · min⁻¹ x 0.80) + 60 beats · min⁻¹ = 172 beats · min⁻¹
Training Zone = 144 – 172 beats · min⁻¹

Enter the predicted max heart rate and resting heart rate of the subject from Step 2 and calculate the Target Heart Rate Zone using the intensities provided.

Max HR – Resting HR = Heart Rate Reserve

_____ Max HR – _____ Resting Heart Rate = _____ Heart Rate Reserve

Record Value _____

_____ Heart Rate Reserve × (.60) + _____ Resting Heart Rate = _____ Target Heart Rate Zone (L)

Record Value _____ **THRZ (L)**

_____ Heart Rate Reserve × (.80) + _____ Resting Heart Rate = _____ Target Heart Rate Zone (H)

Record Value _____ **THRZ (H)**

Step 5 Record the target heart rate zone _____ to _____ beats/min

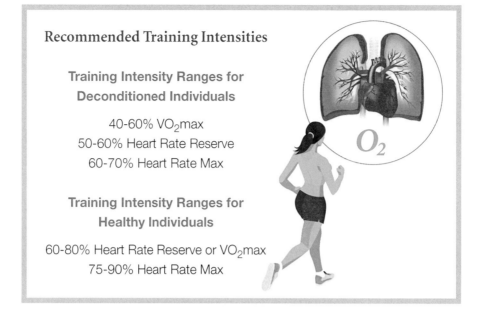

Recommended Training Intensities

Training Intensity Ranges for Deconditioned Individuals

40-60% VO$_2$max
50-60% Heart Rate Reserve
60-70% Heart Rate Max

Training Intensity Ranges for Healthy Individuals

60-80% Heart Rate Reserve or VO$_2$max
75-90% Heart Rate Max

Activity 2 Converting METs to Kcals

Your textbook explains how energy expenditure can be expressed in several different ways. The five most common expressions of energy include:

- **VO$_2$ (L • min^{-1})**
- **VO$_2$ (ml • kg^{-1} • min^{-1})**
- **METs**
- **Kcal • min^{-1}**
- **Kcal • kg^{-1} • hr^{-1}**

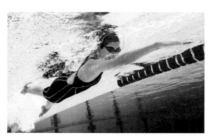

It should be noted that the expression either reflects a measure of oxygen or calories. For every liter of oxygen used by the body, there is a caloric value associated with it. The exact caloric expenditure is dependent on the energy used to fuel the metabolic requirements of the body (i.e., breakdown of fat, protein, or carbohydrates). This is expressed as the Respiratory Quotient (RQ). The RQ is used to separate the inherent differences in the chemical composition of carbohydrates, lipids, and proteins. Different amounts of oxygen are needed to oxidize carbon and hydrogen atoms to carbon dioxide and water. The RQ value for carbohydrates is 1.0 providing the most efficient energy. The RQ value for lipids is 0.7, while protein is 0.82. A mixed use of energy is valued at 0.825. There is a net caloric expenditure of 5, 4.7, and 4.8 Kcal/L for carbohydrates, fat, and protein, respectively. Since it cannot be determined how the energy is being derived without calculating the subject's Respiratory Exchange Ratio (R), the value of 5 Kcal/L of oxygen has been universally accepted as the caloric equivalent for oxygen utilization.

Identifying the oxygen demand of an activity allows the activity to reflect a caloric requirement. The two main components for calculating the caloric cost of an activity are recognizing that for every liter of O$_2$ used approximately 5 calories are expended and that 1 MET is equal to 3.5 ml/kg/min. Scientists have been able to assign a MET intensity to most activities by measuring the oxygen used during their performance. Once the MET value of the activity is known for a given intensity, the caloric expenditure can be derived by factoring in the weight of the individual and the duration of time it is performed. This is the same method used by cardiovascular equipment to identify the calories expended when using the machine.

METs

Expressed as $3.5 \text{ ml} \cdot \text{kg}^{-1} \cdot \text{min}^{-1}$	Minutes reflect time of activity	Kilograms represent body weight	Milliliters identify the O_2 used

Sample Subject:

220 lb. man, 30 minutes using a 10 MET activity

Calculating METs from VO$_2$

$VO_2 = 35 \text{ ml} \cdot \text{kg}^{-1} \cdot \text{min}^{-1}$

Divide VO$_2$ by $3.5 \text{ ml} \cdot \text{kg}^{-1} \cdot \text{min}^{-1}$ (1 MET)

$35 \text{ ml} \cdot \text{kg}^{-1} \cdot \text{min}^{-1} \div 3.5 \text{ ml} \cdot \text{kg}^{-1} \cdot \text{min}^{-1} = 10 \text{ METs}$

Convert ml to L (1 ml = .001 L)

1 ml = .001 L

35 ml = .035 L

Convert pounds to kilograms

1 lb = 2.2 kg

220 lb = 100 kg

Convert liters of O$_2$ to calories

1 L of O$_2$ = 5 kcal

Convert METs to VO$_2$

$10 \text{ METs} = 35 \text{ ml} \cdot \text{kg}^{-1} \cdot \text{min}^{-1}$

Convert VO$_2$ to liters of O$_2$ (1L = 1000 ml)

$35 \text{ ml} \cdot \text{kg}^{-1} \cdot \text{min}^{-1} = .035 \text{ L} \cdot \text{kg}^{-1} \cdot \text{min}^{-1}$

Multiply by kilograms of body weight

$.035 \text{ L} \cdot \text{kg}^{-1} \cdot \text{min}^{-1} \times 100 \text{ kg} = 3.5 \text{ L} \cdot \text{min}^{-1}$

Convert L · min^{-1} to calories

$3.5 \text{ L} \cdot \text{min}^{-1} \times 5 \text{ kcal} = 17.5 \text{ kcal} \cdot \text{min}^{-1}$

Multiply by minutes of activity

$17.5 \text{ kcal} \cdot \text{min}^{-1} \times 30 \text{ minutes} = 525 \text{ kcal total expenditure}$

Procedures

At rest the body uses 3.5 ml/kg/min or 1 MET. The following example demonstrates the conversion of METs into calories at rest. The value only accounts for the oxygen requirement of inactive tissue. It does not reflect eating, digestion, moving, or any other daily requirements that are calculated for daily need. After reviewing the formula, calculate your own metabolic rate using the MET energy conversion equation.

Example

Calculate the caloric expenditure of a 155-pound person at rest:

$1 \text{ MET} = 3.5 \text{ ml} \cdot \text{kg}^{-1} \cdot \text{min}^{-1}$

$155 \text{ lb.} \div 2.2 = 70.5 \text{ kg}$

$70.5 \text{ kg} \times 3.5 \text{ ml} \cdot \text{kg}^{-1} \cdot \text{min}^{-1} = 246.75 \text{ ml} \cdot \text{min}^{-1}$

$246.75 \text{ ml} \cdot \text{min}^{-1} \times .001 \text{ L/ml} = 0.24675 \text{ L} \cdot \text{min}^{-1}$

$0.24675 \text{ L} \cdot \text{min}^{-1} \times 5 \text{ kcal} \cdot \text{L}^{-1} = 1.23375 \text{ kcal} \cdot \text{min}^{-1}$

$1.23375 \text{ kcal} \cdot \text{min}^{-1} \times 60 \text{ min} \cdot \text{hour}^{-1} = 74 \text{ kcal} \cdot \text{hour}^{-1}$

$74 \text{ kcal} \cdot \text{hour}^{-1} \times 24 \text{ hours} \cdot \text{day}^{-1} = 1776 \text{ kcal} \cdot \text{day}^{-1}$

In the spaces provided, calculate your personal caloric expenditure at rest.

Activity oxygen requirement = 1 MET or 3.5 ml • kg^{-1} • min^{-1}

Step 1   Divide your bodyweight in pounds by 2.2 to get bodyweight in kilograms

_____ lbs. ÷ 2.2 = _____ kg

Step 2   Multiply bodyweight in kilograms by 1 MET to get milliliters of oxygen used per minute

_____ kg × 3.5 ml • kg^{-1} • min^{-1} = _____ ml • min^{-1}

Step 3   Convert milliliters of oxygen per minute to liters of oxygen per minute

_____ ml • min^{-1} × .001 = _____ L • min^{-1}

Step 4   Multiply liters of oxygen by 5 calories per liter to get calories expended per minute

_____ L • min^{-1} × 5 kcal • L^{-1} = _____ kcal • min^{-1}

Step 5   Multiply calories per minute by the minutes in an hour to get calories expended per hour

_____ kcal • min^{-1} × 60 min • hour^{-1} = _____ kcal • hour^{-1}

Step 6   Multiply calories per hour by 24 hours to get calories expended per day

_____ kcal • hour^{-1} × 24 hours • day^{-1} = _____ kcal • day^{-1}

Activity 3 **Practical Application of METs Case Study**

Activity Description

As a person goes from a resting state to an active state the metabolic demands increase. The exact metabolic increase is dependent upon the activity performed and the intensity. Using the information that you have learned about oxygen utilization and the relationship it has to caloric expenditure, read through the following case study and perform all designated caloric conversions. This case study will provide you with a better understanding of how to convert the MET intensity of an activity into caloric expenditure, as well as provide you with a better understanding of the relevance of this knowledge.

Procedures

Your client is a 148-pound female who wants to lose body fat. She is training three times per week under your supervision, and at your instruction, has been attempting to expend a minimum of 200 calories per day through sustained physical activity. During a Monday training session, she reports that the only sustained physical activity she was able to do over the weekend was washing her car (3.5 METs) for one hour. ***Does this qualify as continuous physical activity and meet your recommendation of a 200-calorie expenditure?***

Step 1 Convert MET intensity to absolute oxygen utilization represented as $ml \cdot kg^{-1} \cdot min^{-1}$.

_____ METS × 3.5 $ml \cdot kg^{-1} \cdot min^{-1}$ = _____ $ml \cdot kg^{-1} \cdot min^{-1}$

Step 2 Convert absolute oxygen utilization to relative oxygen utilization by multiplying the subject's weight in kilograms by the absolute oxygen utilization value from Step 2. Remember to first divide her weight in pounds by 2.2 to convert to kilograms.

_____ ~~kg~~ × _____ $ml \cdot$ ~~kg^{-1}~~ $\cdot min^{-1}$ = _____ $ml \cdot min^{-1}$

Step 3 Convert $ml \cdot min^{-1}$ to $L \cdot min^{-1}$ by multiplying by .001.

_____ $ml \cdot min^{-1}$ × .001 = _____ $L \cdot min^{-1}$

Step 4 Convert the oxygen used in $L \cdot min^{-1}$ from Step 4 to $kcal \cdot min^{-1}$ by multiplying the values from Step 4 by 5 kcals.

_____ ~~L~~ $\cdot min^{-1}$ × 5 $kcal \cdot$ ~~L^{-1}~~ = _____ $kcal \cdot min^{-1}$

Step 5 Multiply $kcal \cdot min^{-1}$ by total number of minutes she reports for the activity.

_____ $kcal \cdot$ ~~min~~$^{-1}$ × _____ ~~min~~ = _____ kcal expended

Does this value meet your recommendations?   Y   or   N

Activity 4 **Establishing Training Zones Based on MET Intensity**

Procedures

Cardiovascular training zones can also be based on MET intensities. The recommended training zone used for VO_2max is 60%-80%. Using the predicted VO_2max from the one mile walk test or 1.5 mile run test (if the applicable lab has been covered), calculate the subject's MET intensity training zones from the results of the submax VO_2 assessment.

Step 1 Record the VO_2max from one of the cardiovascular activities performed in the Cardiorespiratory Fitness Testing Lab.

Predicted (VO_2max) _____ $ml \cdot kg^{-1} \cdot min^{-1}$

Step 2 Divide the VO_2max by 1 MET.

VO_2max $\div 3.5$ $ml \cdot kg^{-1} \cdot min^{-1}$ = _____ Max MET Value

Record Max MET Value _____

Step 3 Calculate the MET Training Zone using 60%-80% intensity.

Max MET Value _____ $\times 60\%$ = _____

Max MET Value _____ $\times 80\%$ = _____

MET Training Zone = _____ to _____

Step 4 Providing MET Intensity Training Zones means very little for practical implementation and tracking. Therefore, the MET intensities must be converted into Target Heart Rate Zones. Determine the Heart Rate that reflects the MET Training Zone by identifying the steady-state heart rates that occur when exercising at the defined MET intensity. On a cardiovascular machine that provides METs, have the subject exercise at the 60% MET training zone value until steady-state heart rate is attained and record the heart rate value. Increase the MET level to the 80% MET training zone and have the subject exercise until steady-state heart rate is again reached and record the heart rate value.

60% MET Zone _____ $beats \cdot min^{-1}$

80% MET Zone _____ $beats \cdot min^{-1}$

Target Heart Rate Zone _____ $beats \cdot min^{-1}$ to _____ $beats \cdot min^{-1}$

Aerobic Exercise Prescription, Caloric Expenditure, and MET Intensity

Aerobic Exercise Prescription, Caloric Expenditure, and MET Intensity Lab Quiz

1. Consistent aerobic training can increase aerobic capacity (VO_2) by up to _____.

   _____ a. 5-10%
   _____ b. 15-30%
   _____ c. 20-35%
   _____ d. Aerobic training does not increase VO_2

2. Regular aerobic training can promote which of the following changes in the body?

   _____ a. Reduced mitochondrial density
   _____ b. Increased capillary density
   _____ c. Reduced aerobic enzyme activity due to improved efficiency
   _____ d. All of the above

3. Using the traditional heart rate max formula, a 35-year-old male would have a maximal heart rate of:

   _____ a. 160 bpm
   _____ b. 185 bpm
   _____ c. 200 bpm
   _____ d. 205 bpm

4. The standard deviation for the maximal heart rate formula is _____.

   _____ a. 10-12 bpm
   _____ b. 7-10 bpm
   _____ c. 3-7 bpm
   _____ d. 1-3 bpm

5. A 35-year-old male client with a resting heart rate of 72 bpm, who wants to train at 60-80% of their VO_2max would have a heart rate training zone of:

   _____ a. 125-140 bpm
   _____ b. 140-162 bpm
   _____ c. 150-177 bpm
   _____ d. 150-180 bpm

6. A healthy adult should train at _____ of their heart rate max for aerobic fitness improvements.

    _____ a. 40-60%

    _____ b. 60-70%

    _____ c. 60-80%

    _____ d. 75-90%

7. One MET equals:

    _____ a. 2.5 ml/kg/min

    _____ b. 3.0 ml/kg/min

    _____ c. 3.5 ml/kg/min

    _____ d. 4.0 ml/kg/min

8. What does a respiratory quotient estimate?

    _____ a. VO_2max

    _____ b. Anaerobic efficiency

    _____ c. The macronutrients used to fuel metabolic requirements

    _____ d. The increase in respiration when one reaches their lactate threshold

9. For a very deconditioned, obese client, starting at _____ of VO_2max is recommended.

    _____ a. 40-60%

    _____ b. 60-65%

    _____ c. 65-80%

    _____ d. 80-90%

10. What is the limitation of using the maximal heart rate formula on its own for prescribing training intensities?

    _____ a. There is no sex-specific formula

    _____ b. It assumes all clients of the same age possess the same level of fitness

    _____ c. It is an exceedingly difficult calculation to do on the fly

    _____ d. All of the above

Introduction to Strength & Conditioning